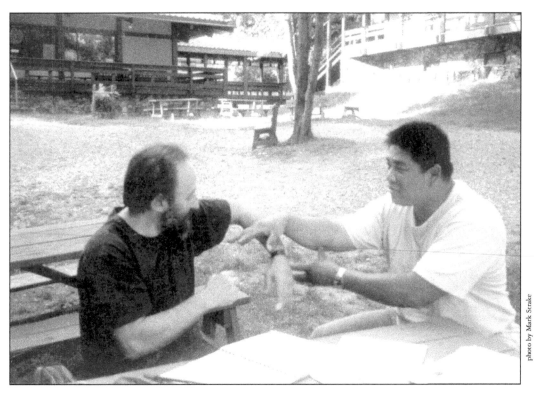

Sam Chin Fan-siong (right) discussing his forthcoming book on I-Liq Ch'uan
with the author (left) at the Chuang Yen Buddhist Monastary in Kent, NY.

Tai Chi Walking

A Low-Impact Path to Better Health

Robert Chuckrow, Ph.D.

Illustrations by the Author

YMAA Publication Center
Boston, Mass. USA

YMAA Publication Center
Main Office
PO Box 480
Wolfeboro, NH 03894
1-800-669-8892 • www.ymaa.com • info@ymaa.com

Copyright ©2002 by Robert Chuckrow, Ph.D.

Edited by Susan Bullowa
Cover design by Katya Popova

ISBN:1-886969-23-x

20200327

Publisher's Cataloging in Publication
(Prepared by Quality Books Inc.)

    Chuckrow, Robert.
        Tai chi walking : a low-impact path to better health
    / Robert Chuckrow --1st ed.

        p. cm.
        Includes bibliographical references and index.
        ISBN 1-886969-23-X
        LCCN: 2002108491

        1. T'ai chi.   I. Title.

    GV504.C48 2002   613.7'148
                      QBI33-598

Disclaimer:
The author and publisher of this material are NOT RESPONSIBLE in any manner whatsoever
for any injury which may occur through reading or following the instructions in this manual.
The activities, physical or otherwise, described in this material may be too strenuous or
danger-ous for some people, and the reader(s) should consult a physician before engaging in
them.

Printed in USA.

Author's Note

Every effort has been made to be accurate and helpful. I have experienced the truth of what I have written here for myself. However, there may be typographical errors or mistakes in content, or some of the content may not be applicable to everyone. It is my wish that the reader exercise skepticism and caution in applying the information and ideas herein. The purpose of any controversial parts of this book is to stimulate the reader's thinking rather than to serve as an ultimate source of information.

The book is sold with the understanding that neither the author nor publisher is engaged in rendering medical or other advice. If medical advice or other expert assistance is required, the services of a competent health-care professional should be sought. Therefore, neither the author nor publisher shall be held liable or responsible for any harm to anyone from the direct or indirect application of the knowledge or ideas expressed herein.

Romanization of Chinese Words

This book uses the Wade-Giles romanization system of Chinese to English. There are two other systems currently in use. These are the Pinyin and the Yale systems. The cover of this book presents the Wade-Giles romanization without apostrophes in order to simplify cataloging

Some common conversions:

Wade-Giles	Pinyin	Pronunciation
Ch'i	Qi	chē
Ch'i Kung	Qigong	chē kŭng
Ch'in Na	Qin Na	chĭn nă
Kung Fu	Gongfu	gŏng foo
T'ai Chi Ch'uan	Taijiquan	tī jē chüén

For more information, please refer to *The People's Republic of China: Administrative Atlas*, *The Reform of the Chinese Written Language*, or a contemporary manual of style.

Table of Contents

Mindfulness/Awareness • The T'ai-Chi Symbol (Yin and Yang) • Some Examples of Yin and Yang • Separation of Yin and Yang • Yin and Yang Applied to Food • Yin and Yang of the Human Body • Naturalness • Being in the Moment • Endurance • Centering • Continuity • Precision • Visualization • Timing • Unity (of Purpose) • Spirituality • Independence and Self-Reliance • Emptiness (Non-Attachment) • Non-Action • Non-Intention • Use of Analogy in Chinese Philosophy • Kung Fu • The Tao (or Way)

Improvement of Alignment • Sunlight • Fresh Air • Exercise • Weight Loss • Meditation • Learning, Reinforcing, Practicing, and Internalizing the T'ai-Chi Principles • Vision Improvement

Alignment • Common Alignment Errors and their Specific Consequences • Causes of Alignment Errors • Psychological Impediments to Optimal Alignment • Approaches to Correcting Improper Alignment • Finding the Centers of Your Feet • Gravity • Falling Bodies and "Weightlessness" • Finding Your Center of Gravity • Exercises for Improving Balance • Use of Eyes • Falling • Fear of Falling • Rolling • Our Sense of Rotation • Dizziness • Subduing Dizziness

Newton's First Law • Newton's Second Law • Friction • Rolling Without Slipping • Why Walking is Analogous to Rolling Without Slipping • The Differences Between Walking, Fast Walking, and Running

Conserving Energy While Walking • Feeling the Natural Swing of Your Legs • Looseness of Knees During Walking • Parallelism of Feet During Walking • Walking Like a Cat • Non-Action During Walking • Alternation of Yin and Yang During Walking • Experiments You Can Do While Walking • Fast Walking • Competitive Walking • Stairs • Walking Upstairs • Walking Downstairs • Walking Uphill • Walking Downhill • Walking on Rough or Uneven Ground • Walking on Slippery Surfaces

Meditative Walking • Alternating T'ai-Chi Movements with Walking • Walking as an Aerobic Exercise • Walking Backward • Walking Sideways • Walking in the Dark • Walking Upstairs, Two at a Time • Running Downstairs • Running Downstairs, Two at a Time • Walking Downstairs, Backward • Walking on a Track • Walking on a Treadmill • Walking with Weights

Hard and Soft Vision • What is Meant by "20-20" Vision? • Levels of Improvement • Myopia • Hypermetropia • Eye Exercises • Cheng Man-ch'ing's Eye Rub • A Story • Remember the Following

Acknowledgments

I am grateful to David Ripianzi of YMAA Publication Center, who gave me the idea to write this book and prodded me to do so. I am indebted to my wife, Ruth, for her help, support, and encouragement. I am also grateful to my colleague at Fieldston, William Werner, and my T'ai-Chi student, Les Hadsell, for their encouragement. I sincerely thank Kevin Harrington, Michael DeMaio, and Tom Grupp, whose instruction of Ninja walking, rolling, and ways of negotiating stairs have been of enormous help in clarifying many concepts. I am especially grateful to Elaine Summers, from whom I learned many of the concepts in this book, especially those pertaining to alignment. Her critical reading of the preliminary manuscript and insightful suggestions were enormously valuable. I am thankful to the following people for reading a preliminary manuscript and making many worthwhile suggestions: Dan Charnas, Helen Chuckrow, Ruth Chuckrow, Bill Eng, Linda Herko, Linda Kieves, Marian LeConte, Joe Mennonna, Emily Perry, Richard Rudich, Flora Sanders, Anthony Sciarpelletti, and Barbara Smith.

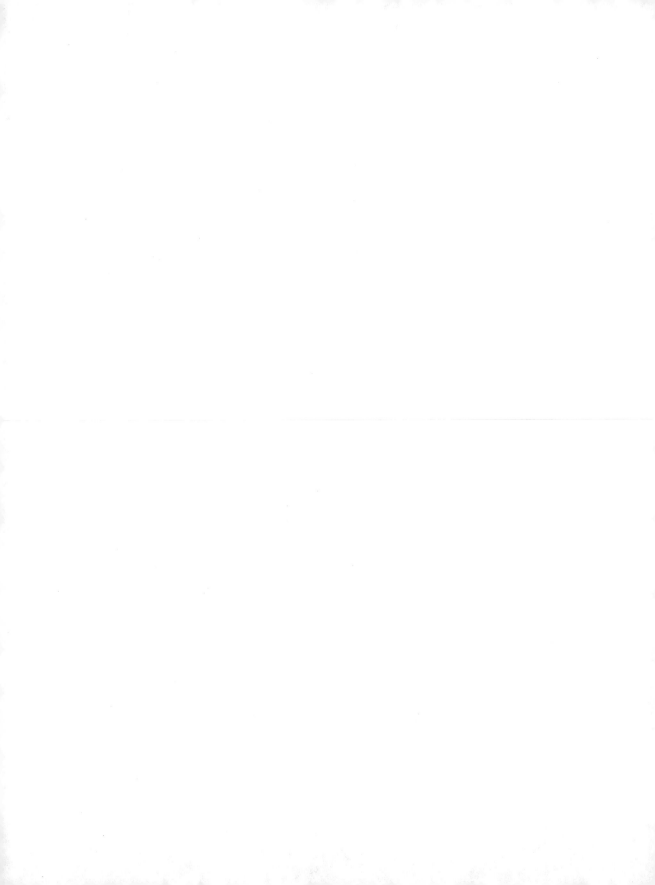

Introduction

Over the years that I have studied T'ai Chi, I have noticed that many practitioners apply the T'ai-Chi principles during formal practice but often not in many other areas of their lives. Principles such as being in the moment, naturalness, continuity, appropriateness of action, and balancing yin and yang seem to evaporate once many practitioners finish their formal daily practice. The most basic aspect of T'ai Chi is that it is all encompassing; it applies to every area of life and living—not just to the realm of practice of the T'ai-Chi forms and push-hands. The T'ai-Chi movements are not ends in themselves but a means of embodying the Taoist and Buddhist precepts in *all* actions.

Walking provides an excellent opportunity for practitioners to augment, refine, and reinforce the T'ai-Chi principles and bridge the gap between T'ai-Chi practice and everyday life. For non-practitioners who apply the concepts in this book, walking can help them to experience some of the T'ai-Chi principles and benefits without formal study of the art.

Walking should be one of the most natural things we do. Most of us have been walking almost all our lives, so we have practiced it considerably. But is something that should be so natural really that way? Did we learn to walk optimally? Can our walking be improved? The answer is that most of us learned to walk in a haphazard way. Wearing clothing, modeling ourselves after others whose movement was inefficient, and having wrong ideas about how our body works are all factors that take their bodily toll in every step we take. Because walking is natural, it can easily be improved to the point where it becomes meditation and improves our health.

During a workshop I took with the late Dr. Moshe Feldenkrais in the early1970s, he asserted that many people are crippled, not from birth defects or sudden traumas but from misconceptions of how their bodies move. I have since seen much evidence that Dr. Feldenkrais' assertion is accurate. In walking, we repeat the same movement many times, and if we have a wrong idea, the harm is multiplied by a large factor.

In this book, I have striven to present facets of walking, an understanding of which will improve your health and enjoyment, lessen your vulnerability to falling, and eliminate harm from faulty body usage. The information in this book should enable T'ai-Chi practitioners to add an important dimension to their practice and daily living.

Many of the concepts discussed in this book have already been treated in depth in an earlier book I wrote on T'ai Chi.[*]

*Robert Chuckrow, *The Tai Chi Book*, YMAA Publication Center, Boston, MA, 1998.

CHAPTER 1

Basic Philosophical Principles

MINDFULNESS/AWARENESS

Mindfulness means that, in all pursuits, the mind is creatively engaged and open. True growth and knowledge result only when you do not blindly accept the opinions of others but are able to see things as they really are. Our bodies are constantly speaking to us (but softly so that they do not become pests). Our inner knowledge (intuition) is constantly percolating through to our awareness. Knowledge from the outside must be confirmed by experiencing it first hand. Every moment is an opportunity to learn, but the mind must be engaged and aware in order to process what is there.

Those who study T'ai Chi develop a constant and deep awareness of everything, both internal and external. Every action—even the smallest movement—causes an effect throughout the whole body. Every thought we have and everything we say to others affects us. An awareness of the effect of each and every thing is absolutely crucial to reaching the highest level of personal growth.

For example, think of how powerful the effects of eating are. One of these effects becomes obvious when a food makes us sick. There is no limit to how much more we can develop our awareness once we are alerted to effects we might otherwise disregard. Food affects every organ and cell in our bodies. Food also affects our minds, and this effect is much more powerful than many people realize.

Because there are so many factors that affect us, it seems almost impossible to unscramble them. For many factors, there can be quite a long time between exposure and effects. This lag ranges from hours to days to weeks to years. That is why it is also necessary to listen to others and be alert to effects that would be very hard to discover on your own.

The feedback of internal messages is always present, but it needs a special way of listening to be heard. One of the purposes of the following chapters is to inculcate in the reader the faculty of listening directly, objectively, and without blindly accepting the many distortions prevalent in others' inappropriate ways of thinking or acting.

THE T'AI-CHI SYMBOL (YIN AND YANG)

The T'ai-Chi* symbol (see Fig. 1-1) represents, among other things, the relationship between yin and yang. The dark part represents yin and the light part represents yang.

Examples of yin and yang, respectively, are soft/hard, inner/outer, down/up, north/south, east/west, cold/hot, dark/light, concave/convex, draining back/springing forth, reflecting/radiating, female/male, contractive/expansive, supportive/extensive, earth/sky, and yielding/taking charge—to name just a few. Of course, the yin component of the T'ai-Chi symbol is at the bottom (earth, supportive, dark, down). Often, when T'ai-Chi symbols are printed in white ink on dark clothing, the dark and light regions are inadvertently reversed. This error is immediately apparent to a T'ai-Chi practitioner.

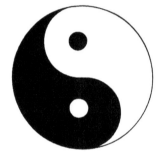

Fig. 1-1. *The T'ai-Chi symbol. The dark part is yin and the light part is yang.*

The shape of the T'ai-Chi symbol represents a circular, cyclic flow of yin into yang and back again. The symbol shown seems to be rotating counterclockwise. The underlying concept of balanced, natural change, without overdoing or underdoing, is considered to apply to actions in *every* aspect of daily life.

Dots of Each Opposite Polarity. Notice that the yin region contains a dot of yang and vice versa. The original T'ai-Chi symbol had no dots. The current South Korean flag (see Fig. 1-2) has the earlier type of symbol, without the dots. The dots have several interpretations. In one interpretation, the dot of yin or yang in its complementary opposite represents the impossibility of anything being completely yin or yang. In another interpretation, each dot represents the inception of the opposite polarity at each extreme half-cycle of yin into yang and back again.

---

*The word Chi in T'ai Chi is pronounced jee, not chee. A similarly spelled, but completely different word, ch'i (with an apostrophe), meaning life force, is pronounced chee.

Continuity. An obvious feature of the T'ai-Chi symbol is its perfect continuity of change. There are no sharp corners—only uniformly changing circular shapes. This continuity implies that we must not allow any gaps in our awareness or any impulsiveness in our actions. Restraint, self-discipline, and awareness of natural cycles are required for eventual appropriate and natural action.

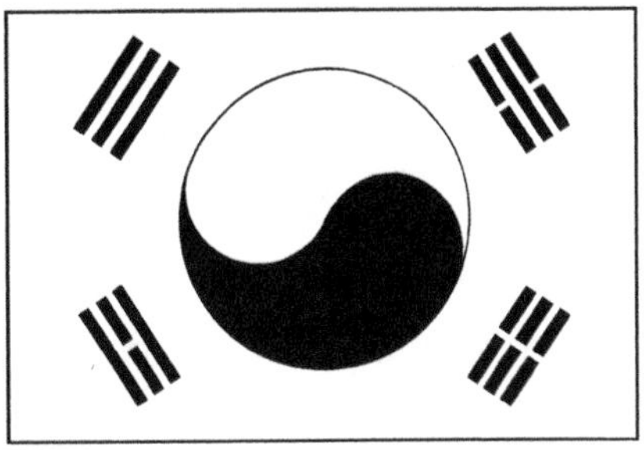

Fig. 1-2. *A depiction of the current South Korean Flag. The colors of the actual flag are dark orange for the white portion of the T'ai-Chi symbol in this figure and bright blue for the black portion. Older versions of this flag have even earlier depictions of T'ai Chi.*

Balance of Yin and Yang. The T'ai-Chi symbol also portrays the *balance* of yin and yang. The symbol is symmetric in each polarity.* This symmetry implies that yin and yang are to be balanced in every action. There are two different ways of interpreting *balanced in every action*. Some practitioners feel that yin and yang do not have to be balanced at each moment as long as an action, as a whole, is balanced. The idea is that balance is achieved as long as yin and yang cycle one into the next to an equal degree. Others maintain that yin and yang must be balanced at each moment. In this interpretation, of course yin and yang cycle periodically, but for each cycle, the inverse cycle must occur *simultaneously*. In both interpretations, yin and yang are to be balanced even if the second interpretation is stricter than the first. A problem is that if attention is not paid to having yin and yang balance at each moment, an imbalance can exist for too long with resulting harm. On the other hand, insisting that yin and yang always be balanced may lead to contriving things to occur unnaturally. The answer is to apply the concept appropriately lest it become self-contradictory.

SOME EXAMPLES OF YIN AND YANG

We do not have to look far to see manifestations of extreme yin or yang becoming its respective opposite. Here are some examples.

(1) Years ago, I had a friend who spent much time muscle building.

*Puzzle: Draw a single line through the T'ai-Chi symbol (the one without the dots) to create two pieces, each with equal shapes and equal amounts of yin and yang.

He was very big and strong (yang). He would lift weights whether or not it hurt, sore muscles or not. At one point, he told me that he had done so much damage to his spine that he could not lift weights any more (yin) and even had difficulty in using a household vacuum cleaner.

(2) Every day, on my way to work, I pass an intersection with a stop sign. Recently an unusually high speed bump was added, ostensibly to slow down traffic in the area. The bump is so high that even when cars go over the bump very slowly, they bounce as if driving over a curb. Some drivers now avoid the bump by going around it, simply crossing over to the other side of the street without even bothering to slow down. Because it is too large, the speed bump actually increases the speed of traffic and creates a more dangerous condition than if it were absent.

(3) When antibiotics were first employed, they were termed "miracle drugs" because they had such a dramatic antibacterial effect. But antibiotics were used indiscriminately, which, according to the United Nations World Health Organization, has created a worldwide health crisis. Now, many diseases are resistant to antibiotics, and there is a whole class of new diseases, which a frivolous use of antibiotics may well have caused. The cycle of yin and yang can be thought to have been in operation here.

SEPARATION OF YIN AND YANG

Separating yin and yang requires knowing the difference between these qualities and then ensuring that each is manifested at the proper time and place and to the right degree. The idea is that yin and yang will each be present in amounts appropriate to the nature of your body and the particular situation. For example, when walking, the weighted foot is yin, and the active foot is yang. However, according to the idea of T'ai Chi, nothing should be completely yang; the stepping foot cannot be allowed to overextend or become stiff, for then it will become yin (weak or dead).

YIN AND YANG APPLIED TO FOOD

Some of the Asian philosophies group foods based on yin and yang. For example, meat (animal flesh) is considered to be yang compared to fruit, which is considered to be yin. Macrobiotics practitioners have even attempted to relate the yin and yang aspects of foods to their mineral composition.* Acid elements (chlorine, phosphorus, sulfur, etc.) are considered to be yin whereas the alkaline elements (magnesium, calcium, sodium, iron, etc.) are considered to be yang. If you compare the Chinese and macrobiotic interpretations, you will find that they differ in many respects and, in some cases, are actually opposite.

Traditional Chinese Medicine is very concerned with the yin/yang balance of the body, and many of the herbs and foods that are prescribed are for adjusting this balance. The subject of yin and yang of food is beyond the scope of this book, and there are many excellent treatments of the subject.†

YIN AND YANG OF THE HUMAN BODY

The concept of yin and yang is all-embracing and applies to the human body as well as everything else. Once you can experience yin and yang of your own body and its relationship to the natural flow of ch'i along the (acupuncture) meridians, you will experience a whole different level of ch'i flow and meaning to the T'ai-Chi movements—and to all actions, for that matter.

As mentioned earlier, yin is supportive, yielding, inactive, contractive, and concave; yang is active, expansive, and convex. In the T'ai-Chi movements, the yin/yang alternations of inactive/active, contractive/expansive, and concave/convex are continually going on. Practicing these changes with in-the-moment mindfulness, relaxation, and continuity will noticeably increase the flow and sensation of ch'i.

NATURALNESS

One of the most basic Taoist precepts is to study and emulate nature. Unfortunately, much of what we see around us seems at odds with nature. Open areas are constantly being paved over where there were once earth, rocks, trees, and animal life. We travel from place to place in cars or other vehicles—sometimes underground. We are surrounded by food that has been sprayed, devitalized, and forced to grow on impoverished soil by using artificial fertilizers. Prepared foods are loaded with preservatives to keep them "fresh," and they are laced with

---

*See Herman Aihara, *Acid and Alkaline*, George Ohsawa Macrobiotic Foundation, Oroville, CA, 1976.

†For a 90-minute-long videotaped introduction to yin and yang and five-element theory applied to food, health, and personality, see Don Ahn, *Power Food: Food for Energy and Healing from the Taoist Tradition*, Ahn Tai Chi Studios, P.O. Box 301 Canal Street Station, New York, NY 10013, 1986.

artificial colors and flavors to make them "appetizing." Many foods that are called *natural* contain highly artificial substances.

The fact that we, as a society, are so divorced from nature in so many respects makes it imperative to compensate by cultivating nature within ourselves.

BEING IN THE MOMENT

Being in the moment does not mean being oblivious to the past and future. It *does* mean that our awareness of what is happening at each moment must not be masked by preconceptions, memories of the past, or goals for the future. Memories and goals should exist in the background to enable our interpretation of the present to be appropriate. If being in the moment meant disregarding the knowledge we have acquired, it would be equivalent to impulsiveness.

> The secret of health for both mind and body is not to mourn for the past, not to worry about the future, or not to anticipate troubles, but to live in the present moment wisely and earnestly.*
>
> —Buddha

ENDURANCE

The T'ai-Chi practitioner knows that persistence rather than goal orientation is the key to long-term progress. Unfortunately, *endurance* also has the connotation of persisting *strenuously* for a limited period of time. The Chinese concept of *kung fu* involves almost the opposite meaning, namely, persisting calmly and patiently *for as long as it takes* to accomplish the task. True endurance requires faith borne of an understanding of time-tested principles and a willingness to persist for an extended period of time.

CENTERING

Centering involves knowing where neutral is in any action and avoiding extremes. We must know how far we are from neutral and from our limits. In movement, centering involves balancing yin and yang by not collapsing or over-extending and not underdoing or over-doing.

Try the following exercise for learning the centered orientation of the forearms and hands: Stand as relaxed as possible, with the center-

---

*Bukkyo Dendo Kyokai (Buddhist Promoting Foundation), *The Teaching of Buddha*, 3-14,4-chome, Shiba, Minato-ku, Tokyo, Japan, T108, 1980, pp. 376–8.

lines of your feet parallel and knees slightly bent. Raise your arms straight out in front of your chest, elbows slightly bent. Now rotate your palms to face upward. If you are as relaxed as possible for that way of standing, you will realize that it takes a certain muscular tension to maintain your hands palm-up. Next, slowly relax this tension, letting your hands rotate until they reach the neutral position with your thumbs upward. Now, continue gently rotating your palms until they face downward. You should feel the muscular tension that is needed to maintain the palm-down position. Again, slowly relax the tension, and let your hands rotate until they reach the neutral position again. Slowly lower your arms so that they hang near your thighs. Again, repeat the rotations with your arms hanging.

You may find that, aside from experiencing the neutral position of your forearms and hands, there will be a heightened flow of ch'i. The ch'i is experienced as a tingling, swelling, and pressurized feeling of the hands and forearms.

Here is an exercise for learning centering, taught me by one of my teachers, Sam Chin Fan-siong. Stand as relaxed as possible (sung), with the centerlines of your feet parallel and your knees slightly bent. Raise your arms in front of your chest, palms facing your body. This popular stance, called the "jade belt," is the basis of a variety of Ch'i Kung exercises. Make sure that your arms are relaxed but that their outsides are expanded (p'eng). Also, expand your back. The chest and inner parts of the arms are naturally yin, and the back and the outer parts of the arms are naturally yang. Now move your arms outward as though embracing a ball filling with air. You should experience a sensation of increasing suction (yin) inhibiting the expansion as you move outward (yang). Stop when you feel that you have reached a degree of expansion beyond which your implied strength decreases and the suction is broken. If you were to bring your arms outward past this limit, your chest and the inner surfaces of your arms (the normally yin parts of your body) would become yang, and your back (normally yang) would become yin. Next, let the suction bring your arms inward, still keeping the outward expansion. At a certain point, the suction will be lost, and you will experience a repulsion between your chest and arms. Stop before that point. Move your arms back and forth within the desired range. When the suction and repulsion (yin and yang, respectively) are equal, you have found the centered orientation of your arms. When you reach an extreme at which either yin (contractive) or yang (expansive) is lost, you have passed your limit and your strength becomes reduced.

CONTINUITY

Discontinuity of action implies gaps in our awareness. During such a gap, things just happen to us instead of our determining the outcome. Continuity results from knowledge of the appropriate principles, applied with mindfulness, purpose, and timeliness. We are more susceptible to impulsive actions when we lose objectivity. When impulsiveness becomes our basic mode of interaction, we fall prey to all manner of misfortunes because we have relinquished our say in the outcome of situations.

PRECISION

Being precise means that there is clarity in our understanding of principles that apply to a given situation and that our intent is in accordance with those principles. If we are unclear about the principles that apply to a situation, we will be confused and, therefore, scattered and weak. *Strength of purpose* and *precision* go hand in hand.

VISUALIZATION

Visualization is one of the most important tools that can be used for manifesting principles naturally and spontaneously in our actions. Every voluntary action is first a thought and should involve thoughtfulness at each instant. A relatively large portion of the human brain is devoted to processing visual sense data. Thus, this faculty is a very powerful tool.

TIMING

Optimal timing is essential in everything we do. The complexity of life constantly challenges us to improve our timing. Correct timing often determines whether or not we succeed in human relations, business and financial transactions, or self-defense situations.

My first teacher, Cheng Man-ch'ing (1902–1975) named our T'ai-Chi school in Chinatown, New York City, *Shr Jung Center for Culture and the Arts*. The Chinese words *Shr Jung* can be translated as "seize the moment." By choosing this name, Cheng made proper timing a theme for our practice and, by extension, for our lives.

UNITY (OF PURPOSE)

When we are in duality, we are much more susceptible to momentary ups and downs. We become like a cork floating on water, riding each crest and trough that goes by. In one minute, our spirits are buoyed up by external events, and the next minute they are brought down. Instead, the T'ai-Chi practitioner strives to develop mental and physical stability unaffected by outside changes. Such stability can only come from a unity of purpose born of introspection, mindfulness, meditation, listening, awareness, and application of universal principles.

SPIRITUALITY

Spirituality means understanding and being in harmony with the principles of nature, on which the universe is based. Movement has a great effect on our ability to achieve spirituality. How can we be in harmony with the universe when physical disharmony pervades our movements? To reach our highest mental, physical, and spiritual potential, our bodies must provide a comfortable and healthy home for our minds.

INDEPENDENCE AND SELF-RELIANCE

The study of martial arts not only builds self-knowledge and self-reliance but, by its very nature, also provides the ability to defend one's independence. For these reasons, martial artists have always been among the most independent people, and the study of martial arts has been considered necessary to achieving independence. Those lacking the capacity to endure the rigors of training over many years were usually not attracted to martial arts or left prematurely.

Those of us who practice T'ai Chi for any extended period are attracted to its potential for self-development. We are willing to put in the time and intellectual effort required. The kind of disciplined and mindful process typical of T'ai-Chi practice cannot occur through blind acceptance but, rather, through an attitude of thoughtful questioning and searching. We, as T'ai-Chi practitioners, are in a position to go beyond established ideas and come to an *inner* understanding of the effects of all things.

EMPTINESS (NON-ATTACHMENT)

Emptiness has a special meaning beyond that conveyed in ordinary usage. Here is a partial explanation by Buddha

> *Fundamentally, everyone has a pure and clean mind, but it is usually covered over by the defilement and dust of worldly desires which have arisen from one's circumstances. This defiled mind is not of the essence of one's nature: something has been added, like an intruder or even a guest in the home, but not its host.* [*]
>
> —Buddha

If we are to see things as they really are and act spiritually, we cannot view the world through overpowering emotions and others' opinions, prejudices, misconceptions, distortions, and agendas. We must empty ourselves of our preconceptions and enter each situation with an open mind. That is not to say that we should constantly erase all of our past experience and start afresh. These experiences become part of a reference library that can always be used to enhance but *not mask* the present.

Practice of the T'ai-Chi form inculcates emptying through *sung*, which is a total release of all unnecessary muscular tension without losing the basic structure. Yielding downward to gravity to can be considered to be yin. *P'eng* is the yang counterpart of sung and involves an expansive upward strength that can be very powerful. Cheng Manch'ing made sung a primary emphasis. He was so rooted (deep sung) that, in his later years, he could not be moved by three or more strong people pushing simultaneously against his extended arm (p'eng).

Our muscular tensions are intimately related to our memories of traumas and the part of our identity that has been molded by outside influences. The act of releasing physical tension cannot occur without a corresponding willingness to release mental attachments. Thus by releasing our bodily tensions, we are also paving the way for releasing our wrong thinking and, consequently, becoming mentally open and receptive. Also, the bodily unity attained from practicing sung goes hand in hand with a unity of thought and action.

At this period in history, we are almost constantly deluged with every conceivable way of thinking by the various forms of media and

---

[*]Bukkyo Dendo Kyokai (Buddhist Promoting Foundation), *The Teaching of Buddha*, 3-14,4-chome, Shiba, Minato-ku, Tokyo, Japan, T108, 1980, pp. 134.

modes of communication. We must achieve immunity to negative outside influences as we take advantage of this unprecedented opportunity to attain boundless knowledge from all over the world.

NON-ACTION

Imagine the following situation. I am driving my car on a slippery highway and get into a skid. After fish tailing a bit and nearly hitting the guard rail, I manage to get my car under control. My passengers applaud me and extol my superior driving skills.

Now, imagine the previous situation but with a different turn of events. I am driving along in my car on a slippery highway. In turning the steering wheel, I realize that the wheels have just begun to lose traction. Without hesitating for a moment, I adjust my pressure on the steering wheel and, almost immediately, recover control. My passengers have no awareness that anything has happened. They do not applaud me or extol my superior driving skills.

Finally, imagine still another turn of events. I am driving along in my car on a slippery highway. Having lots of experience in getting into and out of skids, knowing exactly the limits of my car, and taking into account the slippery conditions, I drive in such a manner that my car never gets into a skid. I do this with minimum sacrifice in speed. My passengers and I get where we are going safely, quickly, and uneventfully.

This last case typifies non-action. Non-action does not mean not doing anything—it means doing what needs to be done in the most efficient manner. Non-action is the ultimate limit of accomplishing something by doing less and less.

NON-INTENTION

Just as non-action is not inaction, non-intention is not apathy. Non-intention is similar to what, in spiritual circles, is called the *law of attraction*. The basic idea is that those whose motives are pure, who are devoted to the process of true self-development, and who assist others to develop will attract what they need for their development without their having any particular focus or making any specific effort.

Consider an example of an author who writes and self-publishes a book with the primary motive to improve his own understanding. Non-intention is operating when the author gives copies of his book to others whom he believes may be interested in and benefit from the book's content. A publishing company may then discover that book and offer to publish it. The author may then receive recognition and monetary reward. This unexpected success can be thought of as resulting from non-intention.

USE OF ANALOGY IN CHINESE PHILOSOPHY

The Chinese are very fond of using analogies to present philosophical and other ideas. The advantage of an analogy is that it relates something unknown and mysterious to a tangible experience, thereby creating a feeling of familiarity. Appealing to analogy is, perhaps, a natural outgrowth of the Asian's emphasis on observing and studying nature, which they regard as a manifestation of ultimate truth. The idea is that all truths are fundamentally the same, so the understanding of one truth can be readily transferred to another instead of introducing a new explanation that might be limiting.

KUNG FU

The closest American translation to *Kung Fu* is "persevere and success is assured." In our part of the world, a great many people have the attitude that if immediate success is not attained in an endeavor, one should either give up the effort or get someone else to do it. Historically, Kung Fu is at the root of the Chinese conceptual framework and explains why non-Americanized Chinese students do so well in our schools.

THE TAO (OR WAY)

The *Way* is spelled with a capital *W* because the word *Way* refers to an all-encompassing path of action and development. The T'ai-Chi movements are only a means of attaining what should ultimately be expressed in every realm of life.

Since every situation is different, The Way cannot be completely achieved in one lifetime and must constantly be aspired to. The Way is learned by receiving correct teaching, doing much experimentation (practice), and having pure motives.

CHAPTER 2

Benefits of Correct Walking

IMPROVEMENT OF ALIGNMENT

The feet, ankles, knees, and pelvis are quite susceptible to injury from incorrect alignment. The lower half of the body bears the major portion of the bodily weight, which can produce damaging stresses on improperly aligned joints. This stress is compounded by the leverage of most footwear. Walking involves repetitive actions, which, combined with incorrect alignment, can produce a chronic problem or exacerbate a prior injury. For this reason, it is essential that walking be done in a manner consistent with the physiology of the body. On the other hand, the repetitive nature of walking provides an excellent opportunity to learn and then reinforce correct modes of body usage. This benefit requires both mindfulness and a knowledge of correct alignment. Chapter 3 details basic concepts and associated exercises for attaining optimal alignment.

SUNLIGHT

Walking outdoors provides a beneficial exposure to unfiltered natural sunlight. Of course, we all have heard that negative health consequences can result from too much exposure to sunlight. Excessive sunlight damages the skin and increases the probability of skin cancer. Less known by most people, however, is that insufficient sunlight (1) results in poor calcium assimilation and failing general health, (2) can cause severe psychological depression, and (3) likely contributes to being overweight. Thus it is wise to get an exposure to the sun but not to the point of damage. An excellent article in *Scientific American** should be read for information about the harmful and healing effects of the sun. More will be said about the benefits and hazards of sunlight in the section about sunburn in Chapter 10.

*"Sunburn," *Scientific American 219*, 38 (Jul 1968).

FRESH AIR

These days, fresh air is an elusive commodity in many regions. We breathe the effluvia of industry and the exhaust of automobiles and trucks. Indoors, the air pollution can be just as bad if not worse. By walking in a wooded area, far from traffic and at the right time of day, it is possible to breathe air that has been purified and oxygenated by the surrounding vegetation.

When choosing the best location and time of day for walking, it is important to take automotive and industrial activity into account. I remember driving along the FDR Drive in Manhattan, New York City, during stop-and-go rush-hour traffic and seeing people running alongside the highway, deeply breathing concentrated automotive exhaust. The FDR Drive during rush hour is not the best place to be, let alone run.

EXERCISE

Because walking is natural, safe, repetitive, and aerobic if done fast, it is a beneficial exercise that almost anyone can do. The elimination of unnecessary stress on all parts of the body is a key consideration when there is an injury or weakness that would preclude other more stressful types of movement.

WEIGHT LOSS

Walking at a moderately fast pace or uphill causes the heart rate to rise appreciably above normal. When a higher heart rate is sustained for twenty minutes or longer, the body begins to rely more on burning stored fat for energy and less on glucose. Chapter 12 is entirely devoted to clarifying the role of aerobic exercise in weight loss.

MEDITATION

Those who do sitting meditation would probably not characterize doing the T'ai Chi movements as meditation and certainly would not consider walking as meditation. It should, however, be realized that meditation can take many forms as long as its general theme is *communing with nature directly*. While walking outdoors, you can readily attain a state of mind wherein what enters the senses is experienced directly rather than processed analytically. The odor of freshly oxygenated air emitted by plants and trees, the sensation of your feet treading a dirt path, cloud formations in the sky, your breathing, and the colors and shapes of vegetation and landscape are all examples of things that can be experienced directly.

Of course, this type of meditation is different from sitting meditation, which involves a state of mind that transcends what comes through the physical senses. During sitting meditation, you lose awareness of your body and the physical world in general. In this state, time has no meaning, and emotions evaporate. Moreover, distinctions such as old/young, rich/poor, male/female, and married/single cease to exist.

LEARNING, REINFORCING, PRACTICING, AND INTERNALIZING THE T'AI-CHI PRINCIPLES

Every movement of the T'ai-Chi form must satisfy the underlying principles. These principles apply to any action—mental or physical. It is understood that practice of the form is a precursor to applying T'ai-Chi principles when we interact with situations in daily life.

In indoor T'ai-Chi form practice, the external conditions (gravity, surface of the floor, etc.) are usually constant and stable. However, the movements themselves are highly varied and complex. In daily life, we must deal with all manner of situations and interactions, making appropriate responses extremely difficult.

In walking outdoors, we encounter external conditions that are usually only somewhat unpredictable. Because walking is easy, totally natural, and highly repetitive, it provides an opportunity to observe ourselves and experience aspects of movement that are much harder to achieve in the T'ai-Chi form or in daily life. Thus, applying conscious knowledge of T'ai-Chi principles while walking can enable us to internalize them. Bridging this gap makes it much easier to apply these principles to the T'ai-Chi form and, more importantly, to life situations.

VISION IMPROVEMENT

Walking outdoors provides an excellent opportunity to improve our vision in a number of respects. Many of us spend too much time using close vision for reading and working on computers. The result is eventual loss of the ability to see distant objects. Moreover, habitually using our eyes to see detail is at the expense of our peripheral vision. While walking, we have the opportunity to see a panorama of objects at a variety of distances, and the lack of need to see detail allows us to open up our processing of peripheral sense data.

Because clear vision is so important and the potential to improve it is so great, a whole chapter (Chapter 7) is devoted to it.

CHAPTER 3

Alignment, Balance, and Falling

ALIGNMENT

Alignment refers to the way the axes of the bones line up. Correct alignment is essential for (1) avoiding damaging pressure on the weaker parts of joints and (2) avoiding shear stress* on the ligaments, (3) lowering susceptibility to acute (sudden) injury, (4) balance, and (5) mobilization of strength. These five factors are discussed next.

(1) When the bones do not line up properly, compressive stress is placed on the outer parts of the joint where the cartilage is thin and cannot withstand that stress. Over time, the compressive stress can damage the cartilage of the joint and increase the potential for arthritis.

(2) Misalignment places a shear stress on the ligaments, which are bands of fibrous tissue that hold the joint together. Over time, the shear stress can cause chronic pain and weakness.

(3) When joints are habitually displaced from their centered alignment, the likelihood of a sprain (stretching or tearing of ligaments resulting from a sudden external stress) is vastly increased.

(4) Balance depends on the manner in which the body is supported in stable equilibrium. Equilibrium is most stable when the supporting forces are transmitted along the bones instead of at angles to the bones. Optimal alignment of the bones, therefore, occurs when they line up with the supporting forces.

(5) The strength of the body depends on correct alignment. If the alignment is off, when you exert force, the poorly aligned parts buckle instead of conducting the force along a line. The buckling not only weakens the body but also threatens to injure it. The result is a limitation of strength.

It should be noted that poor alignment requires a dependence upon

---

*Shear stress occurs when two opposite, slightly displaced forces are applied, as in a pair of scissors.

muscles not designed to support the body. Often, these inappropriately used muscles become overdeveloped, and the appropriate but unused muscles atrophy.

COMMON ALIGNMENT ERRORS AND THEIR SPECIFIC CONSEQUENCES

The most common errors in alignment are (1) forcing the knees backward (hyperextending), (2) flattening the arches, and (3) driving the knees inward (pronating). Each of these errors will be described below.

Hyperextending the knees. *Hyperextend* means to extend beyond the natural range of motion. Hyperextended knees and elbows are very commonly seen

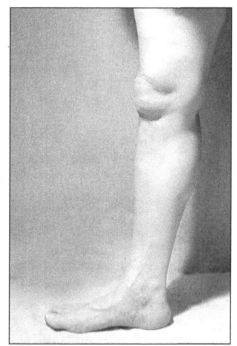

Fig. 3-1. *Hyperextended knee.*

alignment defects (see Fig. 3-1). One of the most basic concepts of T'ai Chi is not to over-extend any limb or lock any joint. Once a joint is hyperextended, it is locked at the very end of its range of motion, and a little tap can cause injury. Moreover, when a joint of a limb is hyperextended, it loses movement options—a defect when it comes to self-protection.

When a knee joint is locked, the above disadvantages certainly apply. However, the knees are subject to most of the weight of the body, and a hyperextended knee experiences a large degree of compression of cartilage at its fragile outer edge rather than on the center, where it is thicker and stronger.

The habit of hyperextending knees is relatively easy to eliminate by merely becoming aware of the problem and abstaining from doing it. A number of students who have come to me with chronic knee pain have experienced dramatic relief after a week of merely abstaining from hyperextending their knees.

Flattening the arches. Many people habitually flattened arches flatten their arches so that the weight distribution is incorrectly centered toward the inside of each foot (see Fig. 3-2). The wear pattern on the soles of the author's shoes in Fig. 3-3 shows the correct distribution of pressure on the soles of his feet. The pressure is mainly distributed over the balls, heels, and outer edges of the feet, with the arches having no pressure at all.

Pronating the knees.
Flattening the arches can cause pronated knees. Or, pronating the knees can cause flattened arches. In fact, it is unusual for the knees to be incorrectly aligned if the feet are properly aligned and vice versa. However, both misalignments can result from an inward wrapping of the thighs as well as a flattening of the arches. In either case, the condition is always harmful and usually self-inflicted (habitual).

Flattening the arches and pronating the knees can cause the following problems:

(i) An inordinately large pressure is exerted on the first (inner-most) metatarsal. The metatarsals are the five bones between the toes and instep of each foot. Too much pressure on the first metatarsal can cause it to enlarge, resulting in a painful condition called *bunions*. The rubbing of the flesh exacerbates this condition in the first metatarsal as the arch collapses

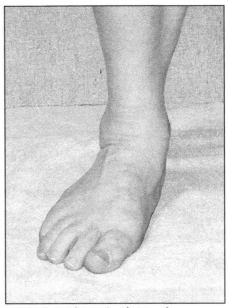

Fig. 3-2. Flattened arch. Note the excessive pressure on the first metatarsal and big toe. Note also the degree to which the ankle is off center.

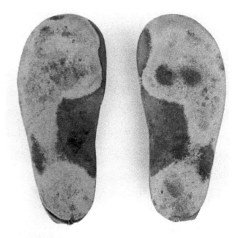

Fig. 3-3. *The wear pattern on the soles of the author's Ute Indian style shoes. He made these shoes without heels or built-in arches. The lighter the region, the greater the wear except for the two dark circles on the sole on the right, where the leather wore through.*

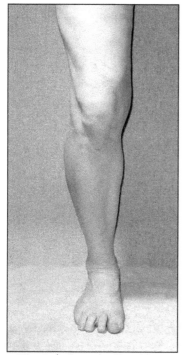 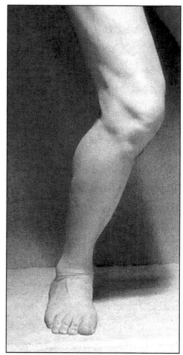

Fig. 3-4. *Correctly aligned knee.*   Fig. 3-5. *Severely pronated knee.*

with each step.

(ii) The ankle joints are displaced from center toward the inside, increasing the likelihood of an ankle sprain.

(iii) The knees are displaced inward from their optimal alignment, placing inordinate pressure on the weaker regions of cartilage and straining the ligaments on the insides of the knees. This incorrect alignment greatly increases the vulnerability to sprained knees.

(iv) The meniscus* of the knee joint can become pinched. This painful condition occurs on the side of the knee opposite to the pronation.

(v) The inside muscles of the calf and thigh are called upon to support weight and become over-developed. The muscles on the other side tend to be underdeveloped (see Fig. 3-6).

CAUSES OF ALIGNMENT ERRORS

Flattening the arches and pronating the knees can arise from combinations of the following factors:

*The *meniscus* of a joint is a thin membrane that encapsulates the joint and contains a lubricating fluid called *synovial fluid.*

Shoes. Babies are born without arches, which form later on. When small children whose arches have not yet formed are given shoes to wear, they are forced to rest what will eventually become the arches of their feet on the built-in arches of the shoes. Also, children angle their feet out to reduce the pressure. It is possible for this experience to lead to a life-long dependence on built-in arches and a habit of angling feet outward.

Heels on shoes lift the backs of the legs, causing the body to tilt forward (see Fig. 3-7). To compensate, the top of the body must lean backward, thus accentuating

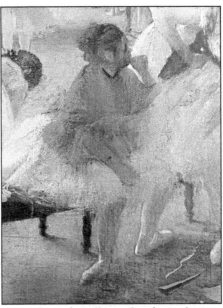

Fig. 3-6. *Ballet pupil with severely pronated knees. From Edgar Degas' painting, "Ballet School."*

the lumbar curve of the spine ("swayback"). More will be said about footwear in Chapter 9.

Copying others. Children learn by observing and copying those around them, especially their parents. Unfortunately, children do not always realize that some things others do should not be copied. Children who copy parents or other adults with bad alignment can spend the rest of their lives with ways of moving that can eventually become crippling. For example, even if women do not wear high-heeled shoes, as youngsters, they saw and may have copied an adult women whose posture was adversely affected by wearing high-heeled shoes.

Societal programming. If you observe people, you will find that many stand with their right feet angled out. Because we live in a right-handed society, people tend to over-emphasize their right sides. Also, young females are taught

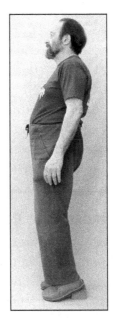

Fig. 3-7. *The effect of heels on shoes. Note how the pelvis is thrust forward, causing the curve of the lower back to be accentuated.*

not to bring their knees apart in public because of its undesirable sexual connotation. This taboo may explain why women tend to pronate more than men.

Effect of being overweight. I have found that those with fallen arches who are overweight find it almost impossible to sustain proper foot alignment. The strength required for maintaining the integrity of the arches increases with the extra weight on the feet. Moreover, being overweight substantially increases the stress on misaligned joints, and greater harm results.

PSYCHOLOGICAL IMPEDIMENTS TO OPTIMAL ALIGNMENT

A person with "fallen arches" or "swayback" and whose relatives are "all the same way" may be reluctant to accept that this problem may result from copying one or both parents' manner of walking and standing. The expression "it runs in my family" too often becomes a barrier to taking responsibility for self-inflicted problems.

It is quite common for many ailments to be blamed on heredity. Of course, heredity determines certain weaknesses, limitations, and the inherent potential functioning or lack of functioning of every cell in our body. However, "fallen arches" and other alignment problems are usually self-inflicted and capable of being reversed.

The first step in changing any habit is recognition that the old way feels natural and a new way feels alien. As you try a new way for a sufficient period of time, your body will begin to know which way is correct. If your mind is open and you are receptive, it will not take long to change for the better. The beauty of this approach is that you will attain true knowledge rather than blindly following others or being a slave to habit. Also, you will be empowered instead of dependent.

APPROACHES TO CORRECTING IMPROPER ALIGNMENT

Physiotherapists and books on biomechanics tend to view improper alignment as resulting from an imbalance of strength and/or length of the muscles involved. Therapy usually involves strengthening some muscles and stretching others.* It is often erroneously assumed that the strength/length imbalance is the cause of the problem and not the result. Sometimes orthotic devices are prescribed to force the alignment to be more correct. Treating the root of a problem is always preferable

---

*See, for example, E. Kreighbaum and K. Barthels, *Biomechanics*, Macmillan Publishing Co., NY, 1990, p. 239.

to and more productive than treating its symptoms.

It is easier for us to blame strength of muscles, genes, and shape of bones for our problems than to take responsibility for how we use our bodies. Bones are aligned or not, based on muscular action. Our muscles are under our direct conscious control, and their degree of tension in every action reflects our concept of how our bodies should move, our emotions, our memories of past emotional and physical traumas, and the particular people whose way of moving we have chosen to emulate.

The approach with the greatest success in reversing alignment problems involves your understanding of the physiology of the parts of your body involved, connecting the way you use your body with the resulting harm, experiencing optimal alignment, and reeducating your use of the affected parts.

A teacher of mine, Elaine Summers, achieves widespread success in working with people who flatten their arches (or have other alignment problems) by employing her system of Kinetic Awareness. First she determines which factors are involved. How people respond to a suggestion of changing their alignment reveals the root of the problem. The problem can be focusing pressure directly in the arches or driving the knees inward. The ankles and the thighs are other possible focuses of inward pressure. The reason for focusing pressure can be psychological or merely having copied a parent or other person when young.

One way to experience the correct alignment of your arches and knees is to achieve the correct distribution of your weight on your feet. The next section describes a method for learning how to center the weight on each foot.

FINDING THE CENTERS OF YOUR FEET

Optimal balance and alignment of the feet, arches, and ankles is most efficiently experienced by becoming aware of the centers of your feet. I learned the following key relationship from Sam Chin Fan-siong:

The distribution of weight on a foot should be centered on the center of that foot.

This relationship needs to be satisfied no matter what the weight distribution between your two feet. For example, in a 70-30 stance (70% on the forward foot and 30% on the rear foot), 70% of your weight is distributed on your forward foot in such a manner that the center of that distribution is located on the center of that foot. A corresponding statement applies to your rear foot.

The following exercise, taught to me by Chin Fan-siong, is useful in locating the centers of your feet: Stand with both feet parallel and comfortably apart, and rock forward and backward. The amplitude of the motion should always be large enough to feel that the center of your weight distribution is alternately forward of and behind what you feel to be the center of each foot. As your sensitivity increases, reduce the amplitude of the excursions, and stop at center. If you do this exercise frequently and mindfully, you will eventually know where the center of your foot is in the forward and rear direction.

To find the center lines of your feet, again stand with the feet parallel. Now alternately bring the knees inward and outward, feeling how the weight shifts from the insides of your feet to the outsides. Again, reduce the excursions until you feel your weight centered on the center lines of your feet.

It is good to alternate the forward and lateral exercises. Do not be surprised if, at first, the centered alignment feels strange. This reaction always accompanies a correction to habitual wrong alignment. Eventually, your body will know and tell you which alignment is valid.

Here is another exercise for improving your awareness of the centers of the feet: Stand with the feet parallel and a comfortable width apart (centers of feet about one-half a pelvis width apart). Try to attain the optimal alignment of the feet just discussed. Bend your knees, and move them in a horizontal circle without moving your feet. Notice that your tibias (shin bones) describe cones with vertices at the ankle joints. Sense the points of the feet below these vertices.

GRAVITY

The force of gravity, which is exerted on our bodies and everything else on the earth, is so commonplace that we take it for granted and give it little thought. However, a basic understanding of gravity is required for stability and falling safely.

Gravity is a force of attraction between every pair of particles in the universe. Because gravity is a weak force (compared to electrical or nuclear forces), it only becomes apparent near an astronomically large mass such as the earth. The gravitational force of the earth on an object is called its *weight*. So far, no one appears to have been able to develop a device that neutralizes gravity or reverses it. Therefore, we experience gravity our entire lives.

The ancient Greeks believed that all things were created in the center of earth and that gravity was the tendency of objects to return to their origin of creation. Aristotle (384–322 B.C.) incorrectly taught that a heavy body falls "faster" than a light one, and this misconception persisted for almost two millennia. By dropping objects of different weights off the leaning tower of Pisa, Galileo (1564–1642) demonstrated that all bodies fall at the same rate. The reason a coin falls faster than a feather is that, for the coin, the retarding force of air resistance is small compared to its weight whereas, for the feather, the retarding force of air resistance is large compared to its weight. However, when a feather and coin are both dropped in a vacuum (no air resistance), they fall at the same rate. Sir Isaac Newton (1642–1727) was able to express the law of gravitation mathematically and, from that, derived that each planet moves in an ellipse with the sun at one focus (the other focus is an inconsequential point). He was able to explain why the tides occur twice every day and why, in the absence of friction, all bodies in a given location fall with the same acceleration near the surface of the earth.

To say that a falling object accelerates means that its speed increases. If the object's speed were decreasing, then we would say it is decelerating. When an object near the earth's surface falls under the action of gravity, it increases its downward speed by 9.8 meters/second every second or, alternatively, 9.8 m/s per second. Thus we say that a freely falling body accelerates downward at a rate of 9.8 m/s². Neglecting air resistance, this acceleration is the same for all objects, near the earth's surface regardless of their weight.*

FALLING BODIES AND "WEIGHTLESSNESS"

When we fall, we experience a sensation of weightlessness, as though gravity were absent. The reason for this effect is as follows.

Imagine that you are in an elevator and the cable breaks, causing the elevator to fall with acceleration 9.8 m/s². Assume further, that you

---

*The acceleration of a falling object due to the gravitational attraction of the earth varies slightly over the surface of the earth as a result of local irregularities and is only approximately equal to 9.8 m/s². When an object falls toward the earth over a large distance, the gravitational attraction is not constant but varies inversely with the square of the distance from the center of the earth.

decide to do an experiment while the elevator is falling, and you release a pencil that you are holding. Because both you and the pencil fall at the same rate, the pencil will "float" in front of you and appear weightless. Next, lift your arms to shoulder level and release them. Your arms will also float in front of you and appear weightless. Of course, neither the pencil nor your arms are really weightless—they just appear to be in your frame of reference, which is accelerating. If they were weightless, they would not fall.

Our main experience with apparent weightlessness is when we fall, during the short period of time that we are accelerating downward. Another experience with the sensation of weightlessness occasionally occurs when we fall asleep. The following is my explanation for people occasionally feeling as though they were falling when drifting off to sleep: When we are asleep, we are cut off from any sensation of our physical body. As we make the transition from wakefulness to sleep, there is an interval of time during which we are disconnecting from feeling our bodies. If this disconnection occurs slightly before wakefulness is lost, you will momentarily experience your body in a "weightless" state. This lack of a sensation of weight is experienced as falling, which may wake you up with a start. This sequence reversal is, for some people, a frequent and quite disturbing occurrence and similar to sequence reversals such as swallowing down the wrong pipe.

FINDING YOUR CENTER OF GRAVITY

The center of gravity of an object is "a center of gravitational attraction; hence, by extension, that point in a body or system of bodies through which the resultant attraction of gravity acts when the body or system of bodies (relatively unchanged in position) is in any position; that point in a body or on which the body can be suspended or poised in equilibrium in any position."*

To achieve optimal balance, it is worthwhile to locate your center of gravity. Because your body is not rigid (e.g., arms and legs can extend or fold), your center of gravity is not always in the same place. However, it is roughly at the *tan t'ien*, which is a region centered about an inch below the navel and one-third of the way from the front of the body to the back. Stand on one foot, achieve a state of sung (discussed in Chapter 1 under "Emptiness"), and move your body all the ways it can go. For this exercise, you can lean forward, backward, and to either

Webster's New International Dictionary, C & C Merriam Company, 2nd Edition.

side. You will find that there will be one point (your center of gravity) within the trunk of your body that is stationary during small movements away from a given alignment.

Once you locate and sensitize yourself to your center of gravity, notice that, for balance and when standing on one foot, your center of gravity is always directly over the center of the weighted foot. Of course, since your body can change its shape, your center of gravity is not always located at the same place in your body.

Then try doing the T'ai-Chi form in the movements of with an awareness of your center of gravity in relation to the centers of your feet. Note that when your weight is 100% on one foot, your center of gravity should be directly above the center of that foot. When your weight distribution is, say 70-30, your center of gravity is directly over the line joining the centers of your two feet, 70% of the way from back to front.

EXERCISES FOR IMPROVING BALANCE

Stand on one foot with your weight properly centered on that foot. Try each and every possible movement slowly so your mind can follow every change. Again, as an experiment, try tilting to one side, forward, or back. Extend your arms and legs throughout their range or turn your body in different directions. Feel your "dynamic" center of gravity always directly over the center of the weighted foot. Next, make sure that the top of your head (pah way*) is directly over your center of gravity while moving. Once you are able to move while balanced, try doing this exercise in the dark or with eyes closed.

You may find it grueling to do this exercise without the visual sense data. However, the improvement in balance you will attain once you open your eyes is well worth any temporary discomfort.

Next, do the T'ai-Chi form with your eyes open, feeling your center of gravity and pah way point always directly above the line joining the centers of your feet. Finally, repeat the form with eyes closed or in the dark.

USE OF EYES

How you use your eyes affects your balance. Try the following three experiments and compare how good your balance is in each case:

(1) Stand on one foot and look at the raised foot while moving it in different ways.

*Pah way is an acupuncture point located at the crown of the head.

(2) Stand on one foot and look at a spot on the wall or a fixed object while moving the raised foot in different ways.

(3) Stand on one foot and soften your vision while moving the raised foot in different ways. Look at nothing in particular, but allow the whole panorama of your peripheral vision to permeate your awareness.

The above experiments are listed in increasing order of improvement of your balance but should be repeated in different sequences. The first experiment demonstrates that looking at your foot makes it hard to visually sense your own movement relative to your surroundings. The second experiment demonstrates that looking at a fixed spot (hard vision hard vision) is better than looking at your foot but not the best way to sense your own movement relative to your surroundings. Using the central field of your vision gives the most detail (unnecessary here) but is not as sensitive to movement as your peripheral vision. The third experiment demonstrates that soft vision enables optimal sensing of your own movement relative to your surroundings.

Next, using soft vision, try doing the sections of the T'ai-Chi form of the movements of requiring the most balance. Then, become aware of the way you use your eyes in daily life (see Chapter 7 for vision exercises).

FALLING

For a youngster, falling may not be much of a problem. For an elderly person, falling can mean spending the last years of life in a wheelchair or even dying prematurely. Because of the serious consequences of falling, elderly people tend to be extremely cautious and limit their movements accordingly.

As we get older, our bones tend to become more brittle—even to the extent that bones can break without much trauma to surrounding tissues. Thus, an elderly person can break a bone without even knowing it. Of course, this encroaching weakness is not solely a result of age; it is mostly the result of the number of years that essential nutrients, exercise, and sunshine have been lacking. Magnesium and a whole group of trace minerals are missing from the average diet, and many factors increase the need for these nutrients. Also, even though much emphasis has been placed on exercise over the past few decades, many people exercise infrequently, improperly, incompletely, or not at all.

Finally, many people are afraid to get any sunlight, and more and more people are usually indoors at their places of work or in school during daylight hours.

Those who study T'ai Chi develop very strong, dense bones, especially in the lower part of their bodies. The stress on the leg bones from doing deep stances encourages the bones to absorb rather than release calcium. Practicing either spirited push-hands or various weapons forms increases bone density in other parts of the body.

A major cause of injuries from falling is that most people do not know how to fall. The most common reaction to a loss of balance is stiffening the body and limbs and, using excessive contractive muscular strength, attempting to thwart the effects of gravity. Harm is then done when a body in such a stiff and unnatural shape hits the ground.

The first level of being able to fall without harm is to partially absorb the force of gravity with successive parts of the body while descending. Less harm will be done if the hands contact the ground with springy tension rather than stiffness. When the force in the hands and lower arms builds up to a dangerous level, the upper arms then take over by contacting the ground. By the time the body is at ground level, it is moving downward so slowly that no harm occurs. Harm to the limbs occurs when the hands—or worse, the fingers—have to absorb the downward momentum of the whole body. Harm to the pelvis or head occurs when (1) the limbs have almost no muscular or skeletal strength or (2) when reaction time is so slow that the body hits the ground before the upper limbs can be brought into play.

The next level of dealing with a fall is to roll. People who study such arts as Ninjutsu (pronounced *ninjits*) are able to fall on rough ground, concrete, or ice without being hurt because they know how to transform the linear, downward motion of their bodies into just the right amount of rotational motion. Thus, successive parts of the body harmlessly contact the ground for only an instant.[*]

Of course, most elderly people cannot and probably should not start to learn to roll. This skill is best developed when the body is resilient and able to recover from mistakes during the learning process. But those who can and do study a martial art such as Ninjutsu, Aikido, Judo, etc., will be much more able to deal with a fall.

[*]For a pictorially augmented treatment of ways of "rebounding" from the ground (*tai-henjutsu*), see Stephen Hayes, *Warrior Ways of Enlightenment*, Ohara Publications, Inc. Santa Clara, CA, 1981, chapter 3).

Over the years, I have had a number of T'ai-Chi students in their late seventies and eighties. I feel that just teaching them to be more aware of all of the different parts of their bodies and how to move those parts independently is one of the most important facets of not getting hurt during a fall. Another beneficial aspect is doing floor exercises, which entail lowering oneself down to the floor and then ascending. Both of these actions plus the movement when lying on the floor help to create a familiarity with both the floor and the changes in the body as it receives the floor.

In our society, we avoid contact with the ground as much as possible. In other parts of the world such as Asia and Africa, people do most of their work on the ground, either squatting or sitting on their heels. Recently, I saw a photograph in *The New York Times* showing Japanese businessmen wearing suits and ties, attaché cases by their sides, squatting and reading newspapers while waiting for a bus.

FEAR OF FALLING

Toddlers usually fall without injury because of their close proximity to the ground and the suppleness of their bodies. As we get older, falling becomes more injurious and embarrassing. Our reluctance to get hurt or be seen as helpless or inept leads us to tend to do everything we can to avoid falling. We tense up, using large amounts of muscular force to regain our balance even after recovery is no longer possible. The result of our tension and inappropriate movement is often an injury that would not have occurred had we yielded to gravity.

ROLLING

Rolling is a specialized way of adapting to the ground without injury during a fall or "throw." Martial arts such as Aikido, Ninjutsu, and Judo emphasize rolling to escape from injury when tripped or forcibly thrown. Rolling can also be used to move quickly downward to evade a sudden attack or as a way of attacking. Rolling seems to be missing from T'ai-Chi Ch'uan,* as taught at present. Traditionally, T'ai-Chi Ch'uan was taught only to those already experienced in other martial arts.

Several years ago, I witnessed an event that prompted me to learn how to roll. I was driving up a very steep hill and saw a young boy on a

---

*The word *Ch'uan* in *T'ai-Chi Ch'uan* literally means fist and refers to the study of T'ai Chi as a martial art.

bicycle coming downhill straight toward me. Because he seemed out of control, I immediately stopped my car, feeling that I had better not be moving if he hit me. When he came about ten feet from the front of my car, he swerved to his left. The front wheel of his bike hit the curb, the back wheel arced up, and the boy shot, head first, over the handlebars and onto the grass between the curb and sidewalk. I was very concerned that he might hit his head on the edge of the sidewalk. Instead, he made contact with the ground with outstretched arms and did a beautiful forward roll. He came up to standing, obviously unharmed, looking visibly embarrassed.

I had mixed feelings. I wanted to tell him that he should have been more careful, but I also was very impressed with his skillful recovery. I maintained a neutral expression on my face, said nothing, and drove off.

Soon afterward, I made up my mind that I would study an art that emphasizes rolling. I found an Aikido class, which I attended for about six months. Unfortunately, that style of Aikido was too punishing to my fifty-eight-year-old body. I then discovered Ninjutsu, which I have continued to study for the past six years with Kevin Harrington and, more recently, with two of his senior students, Michael DeMaio and Tom Grupp. Rolling in this art is practiced primarily for self-protection and is exhilarating for me even though I am now in my mid sixties. Ninja practitioners maintain that fear of receiving the ground restricts you from taking advantage of many critical movement options.

The basic idea of rolling is to transform straight-line motion into rolling without slipping as you contact the ground. Rolling properly requires losing fear of the ground. It is necessary to yield to gravity and and receive the ground naturally.

Ninjutsu, a secret Japanese art until recently, either was strongly influenced by or originated from T'ai-Chi Ch'uan. Many of the concepts, terms, and movements are more than coincidentally similar to those of T'ai-Chi Ch'uan.

Learning rolling is not without danger of severe injury, and, therefore, you should learn it only under the direction of a qualified teacher.

OUR SENSE OF ROTATION

When we move in any direction, we see the background rotating in the opposite direction. Seeing this relative motion gives us a perception of our rotation. There is, however, another mechanism for sensing rotation. Within each ear is a structure consisting of three semicircular canals. Each canal contains liquid and has a patch of hair-like receptors on its inner wall. The planes of these canals are all mutually perpendicular. The purpose of these canals is to sense rotation in any direction—forward, horizontally, and sideways.

When you start turning, say, counterclockwise, the liquid in the horizontally oriented canal tends to remain still because of its inertia. Thus, the liquid in this canal moves clockwise relative to you and, consequently, bends the hairs in a direction opposite to that of your rotation. The bending of the hairs causes neural impulses to be sent to your brain, producing a perception of turning counterclockwise. Similar statements apply to an abrupt turning movement in each of the planes of the three semicircular canals. An abrupt rotation in any direction will produce corresponding amounts of opposite rotation of fluid in each of the canals. Therefore, rotation in any direction is sensed.

DIZZINESS

We become dizzy or experience nausea* when the auditory and visual neural impulses are contradictory to each other or to the actual conditions of turning. Consider the following cases:

Case 1. When you start to turn counterclockwise about a vertical axis, the opposite bending of hairs in your horizontal semicircular canals sends neural impulses to the brain consistent with your turning motion. The visual sense data correspond to the apparent clockwise motion of stationary objects. The neural impulses sent to the brain from both eyes and ears are consistent with your actual turning motion.

Case 2. Now, if you continue to turn counterclockwise, after a while, friction of the fluid with the inner walls of the horizontal semicircular canals causes the liquid to rotate counterclockwise at the same rate as your body, and the hairs assume their neutral position, corresponding to no motion. However, the auditory response contradicts the visual sense data of the apparent clockwise motion of what you know to be stationary objects.

Case 3. Now, if you stop turning, the liquid in your horizontal semicircular canals will continue to turn counterclockwise for a while because of its inertia, and your brain will receive neural messages corre-

---

*One way to reduce nausea is to ingest a small amount of ginger in any form (fresh, crystallized, dried, etc.). Unfortunately, most ginger ale has very little actual ginger.

sponding to your turning clockwise (opposite to the original direction). However, the visual sense data correspond to no motion, which contradicts the auditory neural impulses.

In Case 1, there is no contradiction. You do not get dizzy. If, however, you watch an object that is moving along with you (such as features of a rocking ship on whose deck you are standing or a map you are holding while in a car whose motion is not constant), not only will you get dizzy, but you may experience nausea and even vomit. Thus for continually changing motion such as the rocking of a boat, you should look at a stationary object such as the horizon. Dancers "spot" when doing repeated turns, which means that they hold their gaze on a stationary object in the background as long as possible and then whip their heads around to repeat the cycle.

In Case 2, there is a contradiction; while continuing to turn, you will have the perception that you are standing still and the room is rotating clockwise. This perception is at odds with reality, and you experience dizziness.

In Case 3, you now perceive yourself rotating clockwise—opposite to your original direction of rotation—and you perceive the room to be rotating counterclockwise. This occurrence is perplexing because the fluid rotating counterclockwise and the absence of visual sense data of any opposite motion of the room seem irreconcilable.

The following is an explanation of this unexpected perception: The auditory neural impulses erroneously indicate that you are moving clockwise. The sense data from your eyes should indicate no relative movement of the surroundings, yet you see that relative motion. An observer would notice that your eyes repeatedly dart to the left and then sweep to the right. This involuntary eye movement brings the visual and auditory sense data into accord. Nevertheless, your erroneous sense of relative movement is experienced as dizziness.

There are ramifications of the above perceptual responses for martial arts. That is, giving our opponent a contradictory sensory stimulus will disrupt his balance and impair his judgment. For example, if someone grabs my wrist and I pull away, both the visual and tactile stimuli presented to the opponent are in concord. Thus, he will be able to react effectively. Instead, if I lightly touch his grabbing wrist with my other hand, it will be possible for me to remove my gripped hand with ease.

SUBDUING DIZZINESS

As a high school physics teacher, I frequently demonstrate rotational effects. Of course, it is preferable to involve my own body in such demonstrations. Just after a demonstration of fictitious forces that arise in a rotating frame of reference, I was somewhat dizzy and purposely staggered around for dramatic effect. One of my students, an ice skater, then told me a way to reduce dizziness, saying, "Just jiggle your head side-to-side for a few seconds." I immediately tried her advice, and it worked nicely.

Perhaps the residual, ordered motion of the fluid in the horizontal semicircular canals is disrupted by the jiggling, and the effect of the resulting chaotic motion masks any remaining ordered motion.

CHAPTER 4

The Mechanics and Dynamics of Walking

NEWTON'S FIRST LAW

Stated in its simplest form, Newton's first law (also called *Galileo's principle*) is:

> *In the absence of a force, an object at rest will remain at rest, and an object in motion will remain in motion at constant speed in a straight line.*

This statement may seem to be intuitively false because common experience is that a force is required to keep an object moving. The reason for the required force, however, is that friction is usually present and would slow the object down if we did not continue to exert a force. If there were no friction, once an object were moving, it would take no force to keep it moving.

Actually, we never experience a situation where force is entirely absent because, on the earth, gravity is always present. The earth's gravity even acts on astronauts in a space capsule in orbit around the earth, hundreds of miles above the surface. So it may seem that Newton's first law, which talks about what happens in the absence of any force, is not very useful. However, the wording of Newton's first law can be modified to apply more generally to phenomena by substituting the words *unbalanced force* for the word *force*. That is, in the absence of an *unbalanced force*, an object at rest will remain at rest and an object in motion will remain in motion at constant speed in a straight line. Thus, whenever the forces on an object balance out, the object will either remain at rest or remain in motion at constant speed in a straight line.

Later we will utilize Newton's first law to explain how to walk in a safe and natural manner.

NEWTON'S SECOND LAW

The following is a simplified statement* of Newton's second law:

If an unbalanced force is exerted on an object, its speed will change or it will deviate from motion in a straight line.

It can be seen that this simplified statement of Newton's second law is consistent with his first law.

FRICTION

Over the years that I have taught physics, I have found that few people understand that there are two types of friction: static friction and kinetic friction. The word *static* means *still* and the word *kinetic* means *moving or pertaining to motion.*

Kinetic friction is a force that is always opposite to the motion of an object. Static friction is a little more complicated. Imagine that there is a book on a horizontal surface. If you apply a small horizontal force on the book, the book will remain stationary, but there will be a *static* frictional force of the table surface on the book equal and opposite to the force you apply. This condition is totally consistent with Newton's first law. If you now steadily increase the force you apply on the book, the frictional force will continue to likewise rise. When your force equals the maximum force of static friction, a state of impending slipping occurs. Any higher applied force will cause the book to start slipping.

Once the book starts to slip, kinetic friction comes into play. Unlike the static case, the force of kinetic friction is constant and always less than the maximum force of static friction. That is, if you keep the applied force the same as when the book started to slip, now the applied force will be greater than the frictional force, and the book will accelerate.

The above concepts explain why, when you are driving on ice, once your car's wheels start to slip, traction is noticeably decreased. A similar critical situation occurs while walking on a slippery surface.

ROLLING WITHOUT SLIPPING

We will consider rolling without slipping, which we will show is analogous to walking. Before the wheel was invented, heavy loads were

---

*A more precise statement of Newton's second law is that the net force on a particle equals its mass multiplied by its acceleration, with the direction of the acceleration the same as that of the net force. For a system of particles, the net force on the system equals its total mass multiplied by the acceleration of its center of mass.

moved by placing logs underneath. As soon as the load went past the rearmost log, that log was brought to the front, allowing continuous motion. Even though only a few logs were used, it was as though there were an infinite number of logs, each always ready for support as the load advanced. Later, the wheel and axle was invented, providing continuous rolling and making the use of logs obsolete.

When a wheel rolls without slipping, the point of the wheel in contact with the ground is instantaneously at rest and, therefore, is called *the instantaneous center of rotation.*

When a wheel rolls without slipping, there need not be any frictional force between the wheel and the surface on which it rolls. When a wheel rolls on a horizontal surface, a frictional force only comes into play if the wheel accelerates; in this case, the friction is static rather than kinetic. Kinetic friction appears only if the wheel starts to slip.

WHY WALKING IS ANALOGOUS TO ROLLING WITHOUT SLIPPING

Assume that, momentarily, your left foot is forward. As you walk, your center of gravity advances forward of the left foot, which then becomes the rear foot. Now you need another foot to place under your center of gravity. Your right foot, which no longer supports any weight, is then free to become the forward foot. Thus, the right foot is brought forward. Even though only two feet are employed, it is as though there were an infinite

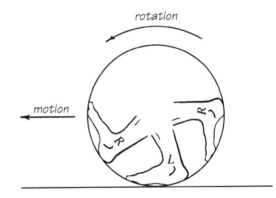

Fig. 4.1. *A representation of walking by likening the succession of contact with the ground of each foot to that of a wheel that rolls without slipping.*

number of feet, each always ready for support as the body advances (see Fig. 4-1). Walking, therefore, is analogous to moving a load with a succession of logs underneath; the use of a succession of logs is mechanically equivalent to a single rolling wheel.

Jarring impact on the body and vulnerability to falling occur whenever walking departs from rolling without slipping. The next chapter details ways of walking in the most stable, continuous, and natural manner.

THE DIFFERENCES BETWEEN WALKING, FAST WALKING, AND RUNNING

When you walk slowly, as soon as your body progresses past your forward foot, your rear foot leaves the ground and moves one stride ahead. The desirable continuity of a sort of rolling motion depends on the ability to bring the rear foot forward in time. However, as you walk faster, it becomes increasingly difficult to bring the rear foot forward in time. At a certain speed, it is easier to spring into the air as you move forward. Now you become airborne long enough to have time to bring the rear foot forward. Now you are running. Running is springing off the forward foot, into the air, as you move forward. Even though running at a certain speed takes a lot more energy than does walking, it is still easier than walking at that speed.

Running is one of the best but most misunderstood aerobic activities. Therefore, running is treated as a separate chapter at the end of this book.

CHAPTER 5

Walking Naturally

Walking should be one of the most natural things we do. It is a basic form of locomotion, innate to almost all land animals. However, walking is highly subject to wrong ideas of how our bodies should move. We tend to ignore the feedback that comes from our bodies, use our movements to draw attention to ourselves, and force our bodies beyond their limits.

CONSERVING ENERGY WHILE WALKING

For many people, the goal of most exercise seems to be to expend as much energy as possible. The recent idea that walking is a good exercise has prompted many to attempt to apply this goal to it. People can be seen walking with weights, using extraneous flailing movements or moving faster than would be natural for a human body. Activities such as swimming, running, and bicycling expend large amounts of energy. Those who are serious about doing these activities usually try to become more, not less efficient at them. The fact that walking is a very efficient form of locomotion hardly justifies making it less efficient. Those who want a more energetic type of exercise such as those just mentioned, should do *those* exercises instead of purposely turning natural movement into unnatural extraneous movement.

FEELING THE NATURAL SWING OF YOUR LEGS

Sit on a table so that your lower legs hang over the edge with your feet not touching the floor. Let your lower legs swing forward and back at their natural rate. Observe one leg at a time in order to experience and capture the feeling of the natural movement that occurs when your legs are totally relaxed.

Next, stand on one leg with the knee of the other leg raised to hip-joint level (with the top of upper leg parallel to the floor). Again let the hanging lower leg swing with its natural frequency, and experience the feeling. Repeat on the other side. Next, walk slowly, reproducing the same feeling as when the legs were hanging. The idea is to sense whether or not the movement of your legs during walking is natural.

Note that as soon as you try to take a larger step than is consistent with the natural swing, two undesirable things occur: 1) unwanted tension and 2) vulnerability of the forward foot skidding forward on its heel. If you habitually take too large a stride, you may not fall when walking on most surfaces, but you will be more likely to fall when you encounter a slippery surface.

Once you have experienced the natural swing of your legs while walking, you can work on achieving the same feeling during stepping while doing the T'ai-Chi form.

LOOSENESS OF KNEES DURING WALKING

By practicing the above exercise, you will realize that the natural swing of your legs is inhibited by stiffness of the knees. As your knees become really loose, the forward motion of your body will result in an effortless, liquid, connected movement of your legs. The feeling will be of walking through knee-deep leaves.

PARALLELISM OF FEET DURING WALKING

In the early days of the colonization of America, Native Americans could easily distinguish their own footprints from those of the Europeans. The Europeans walked with toes pointing outward, whereas the Native Americans walked with feet essentially parallel.

The Native Americans are known for their ability to walk high above the ground on a narrow I-beam. Because of this ability, they were usually hired as bridge-construction workers. This ability is related to a natural use of their bodies and to a lifetime of wearing natural footwear.

Observe the manner in which the leg bones insert into the pelvis, as shown in Fig. 5-1. When feet are parallel or slightly toed out, the axes of the leg bones insert into the pelvis with their axes essentially in the frontal plane.* That is, these axes converge in the frontal plane. To the extent that the feet toe in or out, these axes converge behind or in front of the frontal plane, respectively. When the feet are toed in, the pelvis is pushed backward, and when the feet are toed out, the pelvis is

*For reference purposes, it is valuable to know the three planes of the body. The frontal plane is a plane through the body that divides it into two halves, front and back. The horizontal plane is self-explanatory. The median plane is a plane through the body that divides it into right and left halves. The sagital plane is any plane parallel to the median plane. *Sagital* is named after Sagitarius, the archer (a centaur drawing a bow).

pushed forward (see Fig. 5-2). Thrusting the pelvis forward accentuates the curve of the lower back. As explained in Chapters 3 and 9, heels on shoes also cause the pelvis to be thrust forward, with a consequent accentuation of the curve of the lower back.

The following is an explanation of why walking with feet angled out is disadvantageous: With each step during walking, your center of gravity is ideally above the center of the weighted foot. Angling your feet outward widens the lateral separation of the centers of your feet for a given placement of your heel. The farther apart the centers of your feet, the greater is the side to side shifting of your center of gravity. Widening your stride adds to this effect. Each time your center of gravity changes its speed or its movement from a straight-line path, external and internal forces must be exerted (see Newton's second law, Chapter 4). The external force is usually friction, which, if not available, can cause you to slip and fall. Exerting internal muscular forces expends energy wastefully. Therefore, from the point of view of safety and efficiency, you should walk with both feet as close to parallel and along the same line as possible.

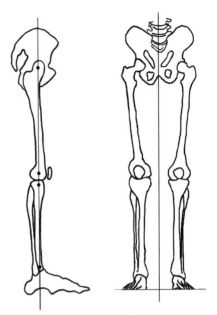

Fig. 5-1. *Left, side view. Right, front view of pelvis.*

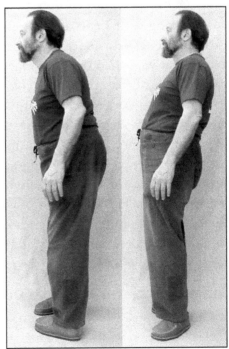

Fig. 5-2. *Exaggerated postural defects resulting from toeing in (left) or out (right).*

Walking Like a Cat

T'ai-Chi footwork is often referred to as "stepping like a cat." This characterization implies that in each step, the foot should first touch the ground for a finite amount of time before any weight is committed (separation of yin and yang). Whereas I soon was able to do the T'ai-Chi form by stepping without committing my weight, I did not believe that it was possible to walk that way in general. I eventually realized that it is not only possible but highly desirable.

If you watch people walk, say at a mall or large store, you will probably observe that most people take steps that are too large. Part of the problem arises because of heels on shoes, which extend the length of each stride. Perhaps another factor is the fast pace of our present society.

If you become content to take smaller steps and lower your body somewhat, you will see that walking can be done in accordance with the T'ai-Chi principle of "stepping like a cat." By walking that way, you are much less likely to fall, and you can achieve a much deeper state of relaxation of your legs as you move.

Non-Action During Walking

Keeping your head at an even keel while walking on level ground. Your body undergoes wasteful up-and-down motion to the extent that your head does not move along a straight line, parallel to the walking surface. Each time you rise, muscular exertion is required. Each time you descend, that energy is lost, requiring additional bodily energy to be expended. Moving vertically negates the main advantage of walking, namely, that of requiring little energy.

Keeping your head moving at uniform rate while walking on level ground or stairs. If you are moving forward by fits and starts, so will your head. The movement of your head is, therefore, a sensitive indicator of the evenness of your bodily movement. Each discontinuity in motion requires unnecessary additional energy and an unnecessary frictional force of your feet on the ground.

Alternation of Yin and Yang During Walking

T'ai Chi practitioners cultivate an awareness of yin and yang and their alternation while practicing the form. Such awareness is fundamental. While doing the T'ai-Chi movements, yin and yang must be balanced in every action and alternately cycle, each into the other.

During one of the classes I had with Cheng Man-ch'ing, he talked about his three "pearls" of wisdom, one of which was to feel his weight transmitted, without obstruction, to the ground through the weighted (yin) leg with every step—not just while doing the form but in daily life.* In order to experience the weighted leg as yin, there must be an openness and liquefaction of the body all the way down to the sole of the weighted foot. Alternatively stated, sung must permeate all the way down to the center of the foot. Achieving sung throughout the trunk of your body has many health benefits and is an important stage of development. However, a higher stage is attained when sung permeates all the way down to the feet.

During walking, T'ai-Chi practitioners can accelerate their progress by experiencing sung, and non-practitioners can cultivate sung without formal practice of the form. Then, with every step you can experience the yin aspect of the weighted leg and the yang aspect of the stepping leg. As you walk, yin and yang will, of course, alternate.

EXPERIMENTS YOU CAN DO WHILE WALKING

Wearing earplugs. As an interesting experiment, try walking on pavement with earplugs, which cut out most external sounds. By listening to the internally transmitted sounds of the impact of your feet, you will then become much more aware of the degree to which you commit your weight. If you walk like a cat, there should be no impact.

Watching your shadow. The next time you walk outdoors in sunlight, notice your shadow moving along the ground. The top of your head should move at a constant rate, with no up-and-down movement.

Maintaining a constant motion when walking up or down stairs. Try pretending that you are on an escalator as you negotiate stairs so that your head maintains an even speed and moves in a constant direction.

Carrying a cup of water. Try walking while holding a cup of water filled to about 1/8 inch below the brim. The steadiness of the water is a sensitive measure of the continuity of your horizontal motion.

Observing your footprints. If you walk in your usual way in snow, soft ground, or a smooth, wet surface, your footprints will reveal much about your walking habits. For example, you can see the length of your

*The other two pearls were staving off the aging process by adhering to the T'ai-Chi principles in every possible action and taking in as much ch'i as possible at every moment.

stride and the degree to which you angle your feet outward. If you walk with bare feet, you will see the extent to which you flatten your arches. The footwear I make has no arches at all. When I walk in shoes on my patio when it is covered with dew, my footprints show no contact of the arch part of the soles with the ground. The soles of my shoes have gradually conformed to the arches of my feet to become raised above the ground (see Fig. 3-3).

FAST WALKING

If you try walking at ever-increasing speed, there will be a point where the energy required to move your rear leg forward sufficiently fast will be so great that it will be easier to run instead. Walking at a brisk pace just below this limit is invigorating, aerobic, and highly beneficial. Many people, however, purposely walk beyond this limiting rate in order to expend extra energy. We have been inculcated with the idea that it is a virtue to expend as much energy as possible. The problem with riding roughshod over a natural limit is that it programs a kind of brutality into the way we treat our bodies in general. Ignoring natural limits and suppressing natural impulses in one realm leads to a consistent pattern of shutting out important messages that are crucial to sense.

I remember walking with my uncle when I was a little boy. He continued to walk even though he was in the process of having a major heart attack. I remember him saying, "I'm just tired. I'll be OK after I rest a bit." We walked all the way to his home, resting every block. Instead, he should have been immediately rushed to a hospital. He was a man who would not listen to his body or, hearing it, refused to give in to its demands. He spent quite a few weeks in the hospital and did not live long afterward.

One of the most important concepts of T'ai Chi is to act in accordance with the nature of our bodies. All of the T'ai-Chi movements take into account the limitations of balance, strength, and extension. In moving, we should become highly attuned to every nuance rather than mercilessly bossing our bodies around.

COMPETITIVE WALKING

It seems that almost every field of human endeavor is eventually turned into a competition. This tendency stems from a preference for egotistical attainment over that of personal growth and physical well being. Our culture places more emphasis on entertainment and excitement from winning than it does on intellectual, creative, or spiritual fulfillment. The fact that walking has the potential to become competitive is no reason to make it so.

STAIRS

A number of years ago I needed to replace a household staircase. Before then, I took stairs for granted and never pondered their dimensions. Of course, I knew that the steeper the stairs, the higher the ratio of rise to tread-width. However, there are clearly defined safety standards for the relationship between the angle of the stringers to the horizontal and the tread and rise dimensions.* After learning the proper way to design my staircase, I became very aware of stairs, especially those constructed improperly.

One frequent problem occurs when the rises are inconsistent. Once you walk up or down a few steps, you unconsciously assume that the remaining steps have the same dimensions. Even a small discrepancy can cause a fall. Another problem stems from a rise too large or small for a given ratio of rise to tread-width. In this case, the dimensions of the stairs are inconsistent with the natural swing of an average foot. This inconsistency can result in your missing a step and falling.

As a high school teacher for the past twenty-eight years, I have had ample opportunity to observe at eye level many hundreds of pairs of teen-age and adult feet treading on stairs. After some thought and trying various ways, I have concluded that the following criteria apply to all the different ways of walking up or down stairs:

(1) The center of gravity of the body is always over the center of the weighted foot.

To the extent that your center of gravity of is not directly over the center of your weighted foot, you are not fully balanced and are that much closer to falling. The more sensitive you are to experiencing any variation of your center of gravity from directly over the center of your weighted foot, the earlier you will recognize the danger of your falling and the easier it will be to recover your balance. Falling on stairs can be much worse than on flat ground.

---

*See, for example, §1910.24 of *Code of Federal Regulations*, Vol. 29, US Government Printing Office, Washington, DC, 1985, p.102.

(2) The center of the foot never extends beyond the stair tread.

To the extent that the center of your foot is beyond the tread on which your foot rests when walking upstairs, you are relying on tension in your foot and friction between your foot and the edge of the tread to keep your foot from slipping off that step. When walking downstairs, having the center of your foot beyond the tread puts you in danger of falling forward, downstairs.

WALKING UPSTAIRS

The safest way of walking upstairs is to have the center of each foot (see Chapter 3 for ways of locating this point) within the outer edge of the stair tread (see Figs. 5-3 and 5-4 for the correct and incorrect ways, respectively). This way prevents the foot from slipping off the tread, which can cause a painful injury to the shin. Once you have practiced walking upstairs this way for a few weeks, you will feel vulnerable doing it any other way.

WALKING DOWNSTAIRS

The same idea of stepping so that the center of gravity of the body is over the center of the foot, which, in turn, is within the stair tread, applies when walking downstairs. Because the momentum of the body is downward, any mistake can lead to slipping and falling downstairs.

The more you bend the knees of the supporting leg, the less the premature commitment of the weight on the stepping foot. Bending the knee of the supporting leg beyond the accustomed degree should be done cautiously. Even if you have strong legs, an unexpected weakness and consequent susceptibility may become evident once you go beyond the accustomed range of motion. You should use a banister to take some of the pressure off your legs while attempting to increase your range of bending. By improving your manner of negotiating stairs, you will also be strengthening your legs.

WALKING UPHILL

When you walk uphill, with each step, your heel is, of course, lower than your toe. This relationship causes a lengthening of the soleus muscle (inner calf), which, in turn, places a tensile stress on the Achilles' tendon. This stress presents a problem for those whose calf muscles and Achilles' tendons are foreshortened. Such foreshortening results from a

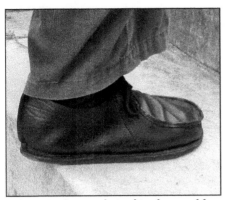

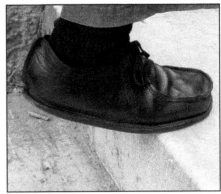

Fig. 5-3. *Correct relationship of center of foot to the edge of the step. Center of foot is within the tread.*

Fig. 5-4. *Incorrect relationship of center of foot to the edge of the step. Center of foot is off the edge.*

number of factors such as wearing shoes with heels and bending forward by lengthening the back muscles rather than the leg muscles.

You can test the length of the muscles and tendons of the backs of the legs as follows: If your shoes have any heels, remove them (the shoes that is), and stand sideways to a mirror. Bend forward at the thigh joints, keeping your heels on the ground and your entire spine, from tailbone to neck, in its natural alignment. You should be able to bend at the thigh joints alone—not from any point of your spine (see Fig. 5-5). Of course, your back will not be exactly straight because your spine has natural curves. You should work on flexibility over a period of time to be able to bend forward increasing amounts (measured by the angle θ without forcing (Caution: Forcing can damage your Achilles' tendon).

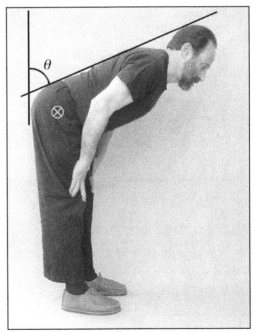

Fig. 5-5. *Bending forward at the thigh joints (marked by theta), keeping the entire spine in its natural alignment and the heels on the ground. The angle θ of your back with the vertical is a measure of the degree of flexibility of your hamstrings and Achilles' tendons.*

The following exercises should gradually increase the range of motion of the muscles of the backs of the legs:

1. Lie on your back, giving in to gravity for a while. Release everything. Bend both knees. Extend one heel to the ceiling, releasing the knee, pelvis, and toes. Concentrate on doing the movement by extending the muscles on the back of the leg rather than contracting the muscles on the front. Then repeat on the other side and alternate an even number of times.

2. Slowly roll onto one side and, using the arms instead of the muscles around the spine, come up to sitting.

3. Come up to a standing position with your upper body, head, and arms hanging down. Allow the weight to shift forward without clenching the toes. After a while, walk the hands out, keeping the heels on the floor as long as possible. When the heels come off the floor, alternately extend each heel to touch the floor. Lower the chest toward the floor. Walk the hands back, and hang. Bend slightly, touch the palms to the floor, and then straighten the legs by lifting the coccyx (tailbone) without pushing the knees backward. *Note: This exercise can be strenuous and should be approached cautiously.*

4. Come up to standing upright by slowly and cautiously by bending the knees, lowering the coccyx, lifting the upper body, and then straightening the legs. Stand for a while, letting the body give into gravity. Try to recapture the heavy feeling you get just after getting up from a hot bath.

WALKING, DOWNHILL

If you walk downhill wearing shoes without heels, when your foot rests on the ground, your heel is higher than the ball of your foot. The upward tilt of the heel of your foot is increased when your shoes have heels. Wearing heels, therefore, limits the steepest hill you can descend while keeping your feet flat.

WALKING ON ROUGH OR UNEVEN GROUND

When you walk on rough or uneven ground, you must lift your feet high enough for them not to become caught on stones, pieces of wood, and other objects lying on the ground. Moreover, it is necessary for your feet to conform to an unpredictably changing surface, which requires forward, backward, and sideways ankle flexibility. If the contour of the ground is extreme, your foot may bend past its natural range, placing your ankle in danger of a sprain. In this case, it is necessary to sense the vulnerability and lessen the stress on the endangered ankle. Protecting your ankle from being sprained may require you to give in to gravity and fall. This is one of the reasons it is important to know how to fall without harm.

WALKING ON SLIPPERY SURFACES

It is easy to slip on level surfaces that are wet, icy, or oily, but once you understand the following basic principles, slipping and falling will be much less likely.

The role of friction. To the extent that your movement is not at a constant rate, you must depend on friction to change your motion. When you walk on a rough surface, friction is available, and no problem usually arises from moving erratically. A slippery surface, however, does not provide friction. If you habitually walk erratically and depend on friction, when you encounter a slippery patch, friction will be absent and you may slip and fall.

You should, therefore, strive to recognize your dependence on friction while walking on all manner of surfaces. Feel the extent to which your movement relies on friction between your shoes and the ground or floor. Then gradually wean yourself from this reliance. Once you are able to minimize a need for friction when walking, you will find that when you do encounter a slippery patch, your body will naturally move without slipping without your even noticing it.

Taking small steps. To the extent you extend your foot beyond its natural range while walking, your center of gravity will be behind the heel of the stepping foot. To the same extent, you will be relying on that much more friction between the heel of the stepping foot and the floor or ground. If you happen to step on a slippery patch, your forward foot will slide forward, and you will start to fall.

It is essential to practice feeling the extent that you overextend in your stepping while walking on all manner of surfaces. Then gradually wean yourself from this reliance.

Sinking your weight. Lowering your center of gravity will noticeably improve your stability. T'ai-Chi practitioners are usually accomplished at achieving a low center of gravity while practicing the form (see sung, as discussed in Chapter 1 under "Emptiness"). However, this ability should be extended to all situations when appropriate.[*] The next time you walk on a slippery surface, notice the stabilizing effect of sinking your weight.

A number of years ago, I was driving my car on a highway a few hours after it had started to snow. As I drove up a steep hill, mine was one of many cars whose wheels just rotated at the rate of the idling engine, with no forward motion of the car. It occurred to me to attempt to redistribute the weight inside the car. I took my attaché case, which was in front of the front seat and moved it to the rear seat. Immediately, the car started to move forward. Next, I inclined my seat to the rear, and the car moved a bit faster. Imagine my glee that elementary physics applied so beautifully.

After that experience, I began experimenting with sinking my weight, not just while walking but also while driving on slippery surfaces. Whereas I know of no principle of physics that would apply, sinking my weight while driving a car seems to make getting into a skid less likely and recovering from one easier. The most probable explanation is that the psychological effect of sinking my weight made me more sensitive to feeling any skidding of the car and more relaxed when dealing with it.

Releasing your pelvis. To the extent that your pelvis, is locked, you will find it difficult to make small but necessary adjustments. T'ai-Chi practitioners can do the form while experimenting with small, relaxed excursions of the pelvis from its centered alignment. Others can do their experimentation while standing or walking.

Feeling your center of gravity relative to the centers of your feet. As you move forward, feel your center of gravity center of gravity moving in relation to the centers of the feet. You can imagine a line joining the centers of the feet and feel any wavering of your center of gravity from directly over this line.

[*]Sung is only one of a number of different states that may be desirable indifferent situations. For example, sung can be considered to embody the element earth, which is associated with the legs and buttocks. Other states discussed in other arts embody water (associated with the lower abdomen), fire (associated with the solar plexus), wind (associated with the chest and heart), and the void (associated with no particular body part). T'ai Chi practitioners have singled out *sung* as the mainstay, perhaps, because this important state is the most difficult to attain. These states are described in more detail in Chapter 2 of Stephen Hayes, *Warrior Ways of Enlightenment*, Ohara Publications, Inc. Santa Clara, CA, 1981

Walking with feet parallel and close together. Earlier in this chapter, we gave anatomical and safety reasons for walking with feet parallel and along the same line. As you walk, you can observe and adjust the extent to which you angle out or widen your stride.

CHAPTER 6

Different Ways of Walking

MEDITATIVE WALKING

You have probably noticed that you experience a deep level of calmness and serenity after doing a round of the T'ai-Chi form. One of the reasons for this calmness is that your mind is engaged in following the principles of natural action as applied to your body, its unified movement, and its relation to gravity, the air, and your physical surroundings. Walking outdoors, with its constantly changing stimuli, can produce a corresponding benefit. That benefit is enhanced when T'ai-Chi principles are applied. As you walk, become aware of your state of relaxation, the natural swing of your legs, the movement of your center of gravity and its relation to the weight distribution on your feet, the softness of your vision, the soothing effects of the sun and air on your skin, and the flow of ch'i through your body. You may become swept into the flow of the moment—experiencing directly instead of characterizing and contriving the events.

The ability to do any complex action naturally, without thinking analytically, is often achieved most efficiently through analytical thinking in the early stages. Therefore, do not expect to experience things on higher levels without first learning from others and practicing and experimenting assiduously. Think of how long it takes to learn just a few movements of the T'ai-Chi form, and then realize how much longer it takes to do these movements effortlessly. The initial process requires attention to detail, struggling with elusive concepts, and time for growth to occur.

ALTERNATING T'AI-CHI MOVEMENTS WITH WALKING

In the early 1970s, when I was a T'ai-Chi beginner, I used to walk to the nearby Brooklyn Botanic Gardens, stroll along the flowered paths until I found a pleasant spot, and then practice my T'ai-Chi movements. People would come close, gape, and invade my space. One man passing by explained to his son in a loud voice, "that man is an exhibitionist." I realized that doing anything out of the ordinary evoked some people's negativity. As time went on, similar experiences led me to find increasingly secluded practice spots—the most secluded spot being my own apartment.

Nowadays, people are used to seeing T'ai Chi done outdoors and know what it is. Still, there is a trade-off of your privacy for a chance to commune with nature.

WALKING AS AN AEROBIC EXERCISE

There is no question that walking fast or uphill causes the heart and breathing rates to increase. As long as you do not walk so fast that your movement becomes unnatural, walking fast or in a hilly area for an extended period has a definite aerobic benefit (see Chapter 12 for a discussion of aerobic exercise and its relationship to weight loss).

WALKING BACKWARD

Walking backward is not an action many of us do for any length of time. However, in an emergency, it may be necessary to do so and crucial to do so for safety. For example, let us say you are walking in a wooded area and you disturb a snake. Not knowing whether the snake is poisonous, you may want to retreat by walking backward. There may be logs, stones, or other objects in your path, and it is important not to trip over them. The way to walk backward safely on unfamiliar ground is to step with the toe, keeping the heel high. As you transfer the weight backward, lowering the heel, you will be able to sense any impediment that might unbalance you. In that case, you can try stepping again, taking the impediment into consideration.

During the time I was a student of Cheng Man-ch'ing, he instructed us to do the backward stepping of "Repulse Monkey" with feet parallel. He claimed to have originated this way of stepping back and said that the lineage of anyone doing "Repulse Monkey" with parallel feet anywhere in the world can be traced to him. Cheng also emphasized that moving backward with the feet parallel opens the front and rear of the body equally. He was referring to the acupuncture meridians and flow of ch'i through the Wu Li gate. However, walking backward with feet parallel also makes sense from the point of view of physiology. If you look at a drawing of the human pelvis and leg bones (Fig. 5-1) or, better, a real or model skeleton, you will see that the leg joints are in their neutral, centered orientation with respect to the pelvis when both feet point forward.

WALKING SIDEWAYS

Sideways walking is required when you need to move in a direction transverse to the direction you are facing. Such a need can arise when you are facing a snake, dog, wild animal, or malevolent person. Walking sideways may also be appropriate when moving in a restricted space.

There are four ways of side-stepping. One way is to step sideways with one foot, shift the weight to that foot, and then bring up the other foot as in the T'ai-Chi movement, "Cloud Hands." The second way involves crossing the empty foot in front of the body, stepping sideways with the other foot, and then repeating the process. The third way is the same as the second except that you cross behind. The fourth way involves stepping in front and behind alternately. Crossing behind causes the body to be slightly turned in the opposite direction of the stepping, crossing in front causes the body to be slightly turned in the same direction of the stepping, and alternating your stepping in front and behind allows the body to alternate its turning. The alternation has the advantage of bringing more of the surroundings into your range of vision.

Just as in the T'ai-Chi form, there should be no premature commitment of the weight during stepping. That is, there should be a short period during which the stepping foot touches the ground without any pressure so that the step can be (a) retracted if the ground cannot support your weight or (b) adjusted to the irregularities of the ground.

WALKING IN THE DARK

It is highly unusual for light to be entirely absent. Usually there is some faint light. It takes about fifteen minutes for the eyes to become totally acclimated to the dark. When I was working on my Ph.D. thesis at New York University during the late 1960s, one of the rooms in which I made spectroscopic measurements was in the basement of the building and could only be entered through a series of three heavy doors that eliminated all light. Preliminary to doing a "run," I would cut spectroscopic plates in half using a glass cutter and align them on the spectroscope in complete darkness. Occasionally, the overhead fluorescent lights would need to be lit during a major adjustment of the equipment. Once my eyes had become acclimated, I could see the lights glowing for hours after they were extinguished.

The eyes are so sensitive to light that you can have a perception of a tiny flash of light from an individual photon. This sensitivity is at least as great as the most sensitive state-of-the-art light-measuring equipment. To give you an idea of how sensitive your eyes are, the energy of barely discernible light entering a dark-acclimated, normal eye, if accumulated for 200,000 years, would only be enough to lift a postage stamp one centimeter.[*]

As less light enters the eyes, color vision and detail begin to diminish. Since the central field of the eye is primarily devoted to sensing detail, central ("hard") vision becomes less effective. Therefore, using "soft," peripheral vision can make a large difference in how well you see in subdued light. Balance, too, is affected.

If you are walking in darkness in a totally unfamiliar area, there is not only danger of falling but of hitting objects, some of which may be at head level. One technique to avoid falling is to sense the ground with a sweeping motion of each stepping foot while balancing on the other. A walking stick can be very useful for sensing the contour of the ground. Moving slowly, continuously, and with the body relaxed will help to reduce the possibility of injury from contacting objects.

It is important to relax while walking in the dark. Unnecessary tension reduces both your sensitivity and your ability to adapt to an unseen object or a discontinuity in walking surface.

WALKING UPSTAIRS, TWO AT A TIME

It is natural to take stairs two at a time when speed is of the essence. Because of the large throw of the foot, it is an easy matter to step noiselessly, heel-first. Be mindful of the strenuousness of this activity.

RUNNING DOWNSTAIRS

Because descending a flight of stairs takes little energy, it is possible to move very fast. The danger is that your momentum may become so

[*]The ears are so sensitive that the energy of barely discernible sound entering the quiet-acclimated, normal ear, if accumulated for 2,000 years, would only be enough to lift a postage stamp one centimeter.

great that your feet cannot move fast enough to keep up with the motion of your body. Be ready to grab the handrail.

RUNNING DOWNSTAIRS, TWO AT A TIME

Whereas it is good to be able to get downstairs fast, taking two at a time is not for everyone. If you are moving fast enough to warrant taking steps two at a time, your downward momentum is so great that any mistake in timing or foot placement can result in a bad fall. Therefore, if you decide to practice taking stairs two at a time, proceed with caution. At first, one hand on a banister is a must. Later, you can have your hand near but not touching the banister. Eventually, you will not need the banister, but even a high degree of skill does not ensure dealing with an unexpected turn of events such as someone switching off the lights at the wrong time.

Another thing to keep in mind is that there will be a larger amount of impact for each step. This jarring effect can be damaging to your ankle joints and Achilles' tendon. Bending the knees more will help but is very strenuous. If you must take the stairs two at a time, recognize the extent to which doing so produces a damaging impact, and maintain the right compromise of tension and springiness of your knees, pelvis, and spine to absorb the shock. This precaution is especially important for absorbing your downward momentum when you reach the landing.

WALKING DOWNSTAIRS, BACKWARD

To descend a ladder or very steep stairs (such as fold-down attic steps), it is safer to walk backward so that your hands can grab the framework. Or, if you are injured or sick or need to be unobserved, you may want to descend ordinary stairs backward.

WALKING ON A TRACK

Walking on a track has certain advantages. The uniformity of the surface is an advantage for those who are frail and worry about falling. Another advantage is the constant proximity of the starting point and possible emergency help. However, the unchanging scene and directionality of motion can become a bit monotonous. If you use a track, it is a good idea to go in the opposite direction for an equal amount of time.

WALKING ON A TREADMILL

The use of various exercise machines has become very popular. One need only go to a fitness club to see a large number of people riding stationary bikes, walking up simultaneously descending stairs, and walking or running on treadmills. It is common to see these people engaged in a number of forms of distraction such as watching television, listening to music, or reading magazines. The main goal is usually to get the heart beating at a certain target rate for a specific amount of time. In such conditions, the mind and body are disconnected, which is not something we need to practice.

Of course, such exercise *is* beneficial, and the presence of many other people with similar motives has a synergistic effect. The unchanging stimulus, however, is boring, as evidenced by the need for additional stimulation. The beauty of walking outdoors is that no equipment is required, and it is free of charge. Fresh air (unfortunately, not always available), natural surroundings, and constantly changing conditions are of tremendous value. Also, outdoors, the lack of necessity for distraction allows walking to be a rich learning experience.

WALKING WITH WEIGHTS

Walking with weights in your hands, raising and lowering them as you go, is an excellent exercise if you want to improve your ability to walk and simultaneously raise and lower weights. Otherwise, there are much better, more natural exercises for developing strength and endurance such as spirited T'ai-Chi push-hands practice, running, swimming, cycling, or using the various exercise machines found in health clubs. The logical way to transport things is to utilize a backpack or cart.

CHAPTER 7

Vision Improvement

Most people think that vision defects can be remedied only by wearing corrective lenses or undergoing laser surgery. The fact is that the majority of vision problems are self-inflicted and stem from the way we use our eyes. Many vision defects can be reversed by reeducating the way you use your eyes. A number of books* describe methods for improving vision—even *beyond* 20-20! Also, it is possible to find practitioners who specialize in "vision education."

This chapter presents some basic concepts and associated exercises. Many of these exercises can be done quite naturally while walking outside.

HARD AND SOFT VISION

A stone-age human being, dressed in modern garb, would go unnoticed in today's world. In fact, sophisticated scientific testing is required to distinguish a fifty-thousand-year-old skeleton from a recent one. The biological and genetic differences between people then and today are minuscule. However, our lives today are radically different in a large number of respects—the food we eat, the way we use our bodies, the use of our brains and nervous systems, and the way we use our eyes.

Instead of looking into the distance and viewing birds, trees, mountains, cloud formations, and stars, we now spend many hours a day using our eyes to see close objects. Reading, if done incorrectly, takes a heavy toll on our ability to see distant objects. Moreover, when we look at details, we tend to use the center of our vision rather than our peripheral vision, which is more suited for detecting movement. Said in another way, we tend to use *hard* rather than *soft* vision.

When walking outdoors, the ambient light is natural instead of originating from incandescent or harsh fluorescent sources, and most objects are distant and part of a panoramic view. Therefore, walking

*See Harold M. Peppard, M.D., *Sight Without Glasses,* Blue Ribbon Books, Inc., Garden City, NY, 1940 or Margaret Darst Corbett, *Help Yourself to Better Sight,* Prentice-Hall, Inc., Englewood Cliffs, NJ, 1949.

outdoors can provide an opportunity to practice a highly beneficial use of the eyes.

WHAT IS MEANT BY "20-20" VISION?

There is a negligible difference between the adjustment of any optical device (here the eye) when it is focused on an object 20 feet away or very far away (*at infinity*). In other words, if you can clearly see objects 20 feet away, then you can see objects that are at any greater distance—even stars, which are light years* away. Thus, 20 feet is taken as a standard for distance viewing, and tests for distance vision are done at 20 feet.† The first number of the pair of numbers characterizing visual acuity is twenty.

The line marked "20" on the standard eye chart is printed with the minimum type size that can be read when viewed 20 feet away by a person with "normal" vision. A person just able to read the 20 line at 20 feet has 20-20 (normal) vision.

The type size of the line marked "30" is the minimum that a person with "normal" vision can read when 30 feet away. Similarly, a person with "normal" vision would have to be 10 feet away to read the line marked "10." And so on. If your vision is 20-40, then your acuity is one-half normal. If your vision is 20-10, then your acuity is twice normal. Of course, 20-20 vision is normal.

LEVELS OF IMPROVEMENT

There are three levels in any endeavor to improve a deteriorating condition. On the first level, deterioration continues but at a lessened rate. On the second level, the deterioration is arrested. On the third level, the deterioration is reversed.

The third level is attainable in most situations. Many experts feel that it is possible for most people to attain at least 20-20 vision.

MYOPIA

Myopia is the technical term for nearsightedness. To understand myopia, it is first necessary to know a little about how the eyes work. The eyes of a healthy twenty-year-old should have a range of focus from about 10 cm. to infinity. That is, there should be no difficulty in seeing

---

*A light year is defined as the distance that light travels in a vacuum in one year. A light year is approximately 6×10^{12} miles.

†Sometimes, when space is limited, the 20-ft. distance is achieved by having subjects view an eye chart, placed behind their heads, through a mirror 10 ft. away.

objects clearly if they are as close as 10 cm. (roughly, 10 cm. = 4 inches) or objects (such as stars) that are essentially an infinite distance away.

When the eye focuses on a close object, there is a natural tensing of its muscles, and when the eye focuses on a distant object, its muscles relax. If we were to look at distant objects as frequently as we look at close objects, there would be no problem. The problem arises because we tend to fixate our vision on close objects such as reading matter for extended periods of time (sometimes hours). When the eyes habitually focus on close objects for excessively long periods of time, there is a gradual loss of the ability of the eye to relax and view distant objects. This defect is called *myopia*, or nearsightedness.

The maximum distance at which objects can be clearly seen is called the *far point*, which, for a normal person, is at infinity but, for a myopic person, can be less than a foot.

The common method of "correcting" myopia is to prescribe eyeglasses with diverging lenses. The image formed by a diverging lens is always on the same side of the lens as the object and closer to the eye than the object (see Fig. 7-1).

Corrective diverging lenses of the appropriate strength bend the rays of objects at infinity to produce an image at the far point. With such lenses, the eyes are then able to clearly focus on distant objects such as stars. The problem is that viewing other objects that are closer than infinity requires the corrected eye to tense to an even greater degree than without the corrective lenses. Thus, with time, the problem grows worse and worse, requiring successively stronger lenses.

One solution is to go without glasses completely. However, as a teacher, it is important for me to see the expressions on my students

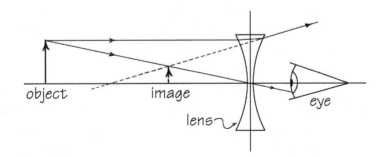

Fig. 7-1. *The effect of a diverging lens on two rays emanating from a distant object. Note that the image is between the lens and the object.*

faces. Moreover, driving a vehicle without the aid of glasses is both illegal and unwise. I have learned that the best compromise is to obtain and use a prescription that is slightly weaker than my "full" prescription but still legal for driving. My vision over the past twenty years has improved to the point where I have reduced my full prescription substantially and require a prescription one-third the strength of the prior one.

Reducing my prescription to one slightly below my full correction is of value because it allows me to most sensitively know whether I am using my eyes correctly. When you succeed in relaxing your vision, there is an immediate consequent improvement in the clarity of what you are viewing, and this change is much more apparent when you are using your eyes just below the threshold of clarity.

HYPERMETROPIA

Hypermetropia (farsightedness) is a condition wherein the eyes cannot focus on near objects. With time and wrong use, the muscles that focus the eyes on nearby objects become weaker. Moreover, the tissues of the eyes become less flexible, requiring more strength of the muscles. Thus, focusing on nearby objects becomes uncomfortable. The result is an avoidance of focusing on nearby objects. Disuse, however, worsens the condition. Eventually, the farsighted person opts for glasses.

Hypermetropia is "corrected" by means of converging ("magnifying") lenses. The best course, however, is to get along without corrective lenses and frequently challenge the eyes by alternately looking at close objects briefly and then resting.

EYE EXERCISES

The following exercises are only a few of the many ways of improving vision that are shown in books or taught by vision-education practitioners. These exercises are designed to re-educate the use of the eyes and undo the effects of prior years of wrong use.

Palming. Palming is considered to be an essential part of vision improvement. It is a way to relax your eyes and, in the process, experience the feeling of soft vision. We tend to misuse and overuse our eyes because of the pace of our modern society and the use of electricity to extend the length of the day. So resting the eye muscles and the neurological processing of images is highly beneficial.

I like to lie on my back while palming, but you may prefer to sit or stand. Start by rubbing your palms together to develop warmth and ch'i. Place your palms over your eyes to create dark warm caves for your eyes. Allow warmth to develop and enjoy the darkness and absence of any need to receive or process visual sense data. While the eyes rest and are bathed in warmth, allow them to relax and relinquish the necessity to seek out images. Think of the eyes as pools of liquid resting in the eye sockets.

Sunning. When you have palmed for about five minutes, do not immediately open your eyes. Instead, keep your eyes gently closed and slowly remove your hands. It is important to abstain from seeking out images as the ambient light (sunlight or any bright light) filters through your closed eyelids. The idea is to sustain the relaxation achieved by palming as you gradually move from darkness to full processing of images. After a few minutes, slowly open your eyes, and allow the images to come into your awareness (soft vision) rather than seeking them out.

Palming and sunning are exercises whose full benefits accrue by capturing the feeling of the exercises and applying that feeling to the way you use your eyes afterward.

Swinging. Swinging is another important exercise, which also has value in teaching balance and body unification. Stand with your feet parallel, about a shoulder width apart or more. Keep your weight midway between the centers of the two feet. Alternately turn your body, from pelvis up, from one side to the other, keeping your head pointed straight ahead. Everything should be relaxed—especially your neck and eyes. You should feel that the turning is propelled from the centers of the feet.

Usually, you keep your body still and turn your head, opposite to the above way of moving. Moving your body with your head still and neck relaxed is very restful and beneficial. For one thing, it enables you to practice soft vision during relative movement of the head and body.

Another version of swinging involves letting your head turn with the body, allowing the changing visual information to enter the eyes through soft vision.

Moving Eyes in all Directions. Moving your eyes in different directions involves moving the muscles of the eyes through their full range. This movement tones the muscles and brings oxygenated blood to the eyes. Since glasses and contact lenses inhibit the range of movement of the eyes, those who use corrective lenses especially need this exercise.

Alternately looking at close and far objects. Alternating looking at close objects and far objects without straining is the basis of most eye exercises. Much of the way we use our eyes involves focusing at a constant distance. The accompanying muscular fixation cuts off blood and oxygen to the eyes, and the tension required tends to linger afterward. Periodic movement is required to reverse the effects of present and past fixations of vision and to teach better use of the eyes.

Activating your peripheral vision. The major part of peripheral vision is mental rather than physical. Whereas visual stimuli affect the retina of the eye uniformly, the processing of those stimuli can be highly selective. We can choose to disregard the peripheral stimuli and pay attention only to the central stimuli. Being mindful of the peripheral information while walking is protective and an excellent way of learning to use your eyes more naturally.

Using "Magic Eye" Pictures.*** For many years, I have had a vision disorder, called *a vertical phoria*. This disorder is like double vision but in a vertical direction. Until recently, when I looked at a single, small object, I saw two identical objects, one slightly above the other. A few years ago, my phoria became noticeably worse, requiring me to close one eye in order to read or to use a computer. Habitually closing my left eye or ignoring what came into it resulted in my seeing almost nothing when I tried to use that eye alone.

On the one hand, I saw that my reaction to the phoria was causing me to lose the sight in my left eye, and on the other hand, I knew that using glasses with prisms to "correct" the phoria was going to eventually make it worse. I therefore set out to design an exercise to overcome the problem. I was familiar with "Magic Eye" pictures, which enable the viewer to see a three-dimensional scene when the picture is viewed in a certain way (see Fig. 7-2). I knew that seeing these pictures requires both eyes to work together equally. I started working daily and saw daily progress.

Knowing that prisms are used to "correct" the phoria, I further strengthened my eyes by orienting prisms in reverse to make it even

*****Marc Grossman, O.D. and Rachel Cooper, *Magic Eye: How to See 3D*, Andrews and McMeel Co., Kansas City, MO, 1995, ISBN 0-8362-0467-0.

harder for me to view the pictures. Today, my phoria is barely noticeable, and I only need to view the "Magic Eye" pictures occasionally (about once every few weeks).

I am convinced that these exercises also have reduced my myopia.

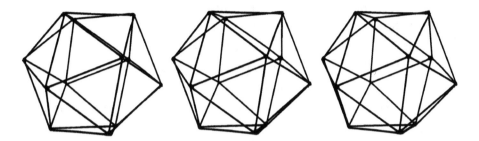

Fig. 7-2. An example of a "3-D" picture created by the author. To view the figure, first mask off the text above and below it. Then place the middle icosahedron as close as possible to your face, at the midpoint between your two eyes. Relax your vision as though you were looking at a distant object. The figure will, of course, be out of focus, but you will now see two icosahedrons. Next, move the figure away (at a comfortable length) from your face until you can see it clearly. If you are successful, you will see four icosahedrons, with the middle two icosahedrons perceived as three-dimensional.

CHENG MAN-CH'ING'S EYE RUB

When I was a beginning student under Cheng Man-ch'ing, he made a special point of showing me a massage for the eyes. The massage does not actually involve any pressure on the eyes but, rather, on the bony ridges of the eye sockets. Start by propping your forefingers against your forehead. Place the first joints (near the nail) of your thumb against the outside corners of your eyes. Move the thumb joints inward along the top of the ridges of the eye sockets, and then move out along the bottoms. Repeat for a total of thirty-six times.

A STORY

About twenty years ago, I had a physics student whose vision was very poor. He wore fairly strong glasses and always seemed to find it hard to look directly toward me. Each time I had a conversation with him, he would move to my side, so that we were at right angles to each other. As I turned to face him, he would simultaneously move to maintain the 90-degree relationship.

After the summer vacation, I noticed that he was not wearing glasses. Now, he faced me head-on, not 90 degrees to the side. I spoke to him about his improved vision. He reminded me that I had discussed vision when we covered optics. I had mentioned that there were professionals who did vision education even though I did not know any practitioner at that time. Over the summer, he had found someone with whom to study. At the end of the summer, his vision was normal. He gave me the name and phone number of the practitioner, Renate Wassell, who worked with him, and I made an appointment with her.

When I arrived after a two-hour drive, Ms. Wassell immediately told me that I must remove my glasses and not ever wear them while in her house. She first had me stand in a specific spot and took out a box of index cards. Each card had a letter or number on it. She held up a card, and I then identified what it said. Then she kept moving farther away, each time showing me a different card to identify. She put down the box when I could not read any additional cards.

Next, we spent about an hour-and-a-half doing various eye exercises alternating with palming and sunning. She then told me to go over to the original card-reading spot, picked up the box of cards, and resumed testing my ability to identify them. I was amazed at how much farther she was able to move away before I again reached the limit of my vision.

When I drove home, I was amazed at how clear things were. I estimated that my eyes had improved by one prescription (0.25 diopters). It was impractical to visit Ms. Wassell regularly as it required four hours of driving. She knew, however, that I would be able to come only a few times and had generously given me the tools to be able to work on my own.

I found that progress was much slower when working on my own. Moreover, when I neglected to do the exercises for a few months, my vision noticeably deteriorated. On the whole, however, I have continued to make progress.

REMEMBER THE FOLLOWING

The basic rule is, *you get good at what you practice, whether it is beneficial or harmful.* Practice soft vision and peripheral vision. Do not fixate your gaze at one distance or in one direction. Do not limit yourself with a goal to attain mere 20-20 vision. Most of us are capable of attaining 20-15 or 20-10 acuity. Even if you have 20-20 or better vision, you can still improve your peripheral vision.

CHAPTER 8

Care of Feet

HYGIENE OF FEET

Walking is such a pleasure when your feet are healthy and comfortable. Unfortunately, feet spend a good part of the day encapsulated in shoes. Thus, they do not get enough oxygenation, ventilation, and beneficial movement. The lack of oxygen is problematic since oxygen inhibits growth of bacteria. Also, feet are close to the dirty, bacteria-dense ground, and perspiration, which evaporates slowly because of insufficient ventilation, becomes a medium for bacterial decomposition. Therefore, feet trapped in shoes for long periods of time tend to be unhealthy, uncomfortable, and foul-smelling.

Washing the feet frequently with soap and may seem like a good idea but is not. Soap is, itself, a medium for bacterial growth. Because soap is alkaline, it disrupts the skin's natural acidity, which inhibits bacterial growth. You may then ask, "How can I keep myself clean without soap?" The answer is multifold:

1. Wash only with pure water and friction. You will find that, unless you step barefooted in a puddle of axle grease, pure water is all that is necessary for optimal hygiene of the skin. However, water alone is insufficient for washing hair. A natural shampoo is recommended for hair.

2. Make sure that everything that touches your feet is immaculately clean. This means that the shower floor, the bath mat, the towel used for your feet, the bathroom scale, the floor of the bathroom, and your socks must all be washed frequently—preferably with a germicidal solution such as household bleach.

3. After taking a bath or shower, it is good to apply hydrogen peroxide (readily obtainable in any supermarket or pharmacy as a 3% solution) to the dry feet, especially between the toes

and at their roots. Hydrogen peroxide both inhibits the growth of bacteria and removes dead skin on which bacteria flourish. Then dry the feet and apply a 70% solution of alcohol. You are probably concerned (as I am) about the toxicity of store-bought rubbing alcohol, which is much more poisonous than a solution of pure ethyl alcohol and water mixed to a 70% concentration. What I do is purchase a bottle of 190-proof (95%) vodka and a bottle of 80-proof (40%) vodka in a liquor store. Remember those mixture problems you used to get for homework in algebra class? Well, here's one: In what proportion should the above two vodkas be mixed to produce 70% vodka? You can check my algebra if you want, but, in the meantime, I get 5 fluid ounces of 80-proof (40%) vodka to 6 fluid ounces of 190-proof (95%) vodka to obtain approximately* 11 fluid ounces 140-proof (70%) vodka. Similarly, the 95% vodka can be diluted to the 70% concentration by adding 5 fluid ounces of water to 14 fluid ounces of 190-proof (95%) vodka to obtain approximately 19 ounces of 140-proof (70%) vodka.

VENTILATION

It is very important to oxygenate the feet and allow perspiration to evaporate whenever possible. The higher the tops of the shoes and the tighter they are, the less air flow there is. It is advisable to remove your shoes whenever possible, even if only for a few minutes. As the perspiration evaporates, your feet will feel cool—a beneficial sign. When your shoes are off, it is a good time to do some foot exercises, as discussed in the section after next.

SOAKING THE FEET

As a wonderful treat for tired feet, try soaking them in warm water to which some salt is added. A dishpan is about the right size and can be reserved for this purpose. You can slowly raise the temperature of the water, but those with a heart conditions should be aware that too high a temperature for too long can put a strain on the heart.

---

*It is interesting that if you carefully measure the total volume of the mixture, it will be slightly less than the sum of the volumes of the two parts. This discrepancy results from the fact that alcohol and water dissolve in each other.

FOOT EXERCISES

Toning and strengthening the muscles of the feet are quite important. The following exercise is best done while lying on your back on the floor. Start by rotating each foot in a circle at the ankle, first clockwise, then counterclockwise, and repeat both directions. Then extend the heels and then the toes, and repeat both actions. Cautiously make a fist with the toes of one foot. Then relax and go to the other foot. Alternate from one foot to the other, each time flexing more strenuously, as the tissues tone up. If you make fists with the toes daily, you will reach the point where you can make as strong a fist with your toes as you can with your fingers. Next, alternately spread and release the toes of both feet. Then alternately tap the heels of the feet against the floor to stimulate the bones and the flow of ch'i. Next, clap the insides of the feet together.

Feel the effect throughout the whole body between each exercise and the next. You should find that these simple exercises will give your feet a new lease on life. Whereas the above routine can be done at any time of the day or night, much benefit is achieved by doing it in the early morning before you get out of bed and put weight on your feet (you can find a way to tap the heels on the floor while lying or sitting on the bed). Later in the day, when the feet have been encased in shoes for a period of time, they will be more susceptible to spasm, and the foot exercises should be done with extra caution.

CALF-STRENGTHENING EXERCISES

Calf muscles are much less susceptible to fatigue and cramps when they are strong and in good tone. Calves can be easily strengthened by the following exercise: Stand on the ball of one foot in a doorway with one hand on each jamb for support. Alternately lift and lower your body, taking the largest possible vertical excursions. The first time, do this exercise very cautiously with very few repetitions—it is quite strenuous. Afterward, shake the foot at the ankle to relieve the tension in the calf.

Try doing the movements of the T'ai-Chi form, keeping your heels always lifted. This method of strengthening the feet and legs was taught to me by Harvey I. Sober, a high-level martial-arts and Ch'i-Kung grandmaster.

FOOT MASSAGE

Most footwear does not permit the full muscular movement of feet. Unless you walk exclusively during warm weather and on soft ground, you probably will not do much walking barefooted. In this case, you will need to wear some sort of footwear, which, over any period of time, will inhibit the natural movement of your feet. The following foot massage will be of much value in toning the feet*

1. While sitting, lift one foot and let it rest on your thigh. Grab the toes with the opposite hand and rotate the whole foot about the ankle fifteen times in one direction (see Fig. 8-1). Then repeat fifteen times in the other direction.

2. Grab the toes with the opposite hand and rotate the whole toe end of the foot, first in one direction and then in the other direction (see Fig. 8-2).

3. Sitting, bend one knee and lift the foot on that side. Reach under the foot with the opposite hand so that the fifth metatarsal is cradled in the hollow of the palm. Then similarly cradle the first metatarsal in the palm of the other hand. Applying moderate pressure, briskly move the hands toward and away from the body in opposite directions. This action will cause the foot to be twisted back and forth (see Fig. 8-3).

4. Grab the big toe between your thumb and forefinger of the hand opposite the foot and crank the toe in a circle. Crank each toe in turn (see Fig. 8-4).

5. Squeeze the sides of the first joint (near the root of the nail) of the big toe between your thumb and forefinger. Roll the joint back and forth in each direction (see Fig. 8-5). Repeat with each toe in turn.

6. Place the outer edge of your extended hand between the big toe and the next. Then massage the space between with a vigorous sawing motion. Repeat for each successive pair of toes (see Fig. 8-6).

7. Dig the nails of fingers into the tips of the toes (see Fig. 8-7).

8. Dig the nails of fingers into the roots of the toes (see Fig. 8-8).

*To learn about a ch'i-meridian-based self massage, see Jacques de Langre, *The First Book of Do-In*, Happiness Press, 1607 North Sierra Bonita Avenue, Hollywood, CA 90046, 1971.

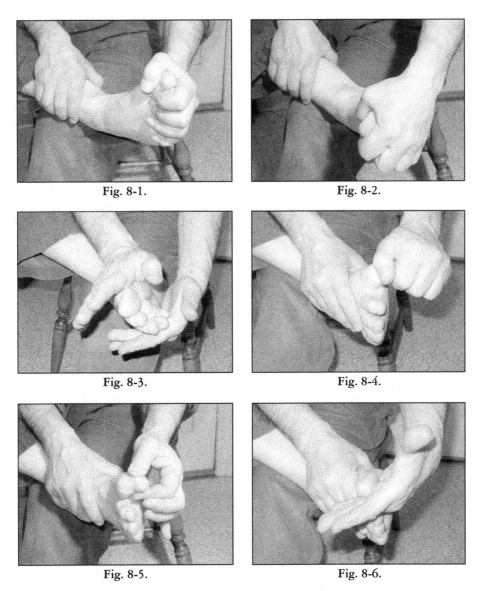

Fig. 8-1.

Fig. 8-2.

Fig. 8-3.

Fig. 8-4.

Fig. 8-5.

Fig. 8-6.

9. Starting at the inner ankle, briskly rub the palm of the hand across the arch toward the little toe and back. Cheng Man-ch'ing taught me this rub and said to do it briskly, twenty-one times in rapid succession to each foot (see Fig. 8-9).

10. End by feeling the yin chuen point ("bubbling well") located on the center of the sole of the foot, just below the ball of the foot.

11–20. Repeat steps 1–10 on the other foot.

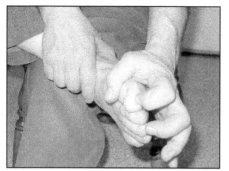

Fig. 8-7.

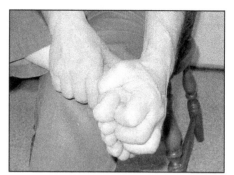

Fig. 8-8.

KICKING TO RELIEVE TENSION

The muscles that move the lower legs are located primarily in the upper legs. Similarly, the muscles that move the feet are located primarily in the lower legs. Thus, tension in one quadriceps* is released by standing on the other leg and loosely kicking the heel of the empty foot forward, pivoting at

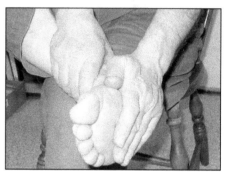

Fig. 8-9.

the knee. Similarly, tension in each calf is released by standing on the foot on the other side and loosely flapping the empty foot.

Cheng Man-ch'ing showed me the heel-kicking exercise during my very first class with him in April, 1970.

---

*The quadriceps is the large muscle of the front of the thigh. The quadriceps extends the leg by its contraction and is considered to have four heads or origins.

Footwear and Clothing

FOOTWEAR

Footwear may well date back seventy-five-thousand years. Footwear from parts of the world that have not been changed by encroaching civilization is usually suited to the weather and terrain. For example, Native American footwear from the high plains had hard soles, which are more difficult to make but are more suited for protection from cactus and hard ground.[*] The ideal footwear is a compromise between protecting the feet and permitting feet their full range of movement. The more protection, the less movement; the more movement, the less protection. George White[†] and Sylvia Granger[‡] give practical designs and instructions for making Native American footwear.

The fact that much modern footwear is designed mainly for appearance results in a disregard for functionality. Moreover, many misconceptions about feet have become generally accepted to the point that few people understand the anatomical function of the feet and the appropriate role of footwear.[§] Unfortunately, most modern footwear reflects these misconceptions.

Short of having footwear custom made or making your own, purchasing commercial footwear is not a bad idea as long as you avoid the pitfalls outlined in this chapter. Many people like to wear cloth Kung-Fu slippers, which are available in some stores at a very reasonable price.[||] This footwear has practically no heels or built-in arches. We will

[*]George M. White, *Craft Manual of the North American Indian Footwear*, George M. White, P.O. Box 365, Ronan, MT 59684, 1969, p. 10.

[†]Ibid.

[‡]Sylvia Granger, How to Make Your Own Moccasins, J.B. Lippincott Company, New York, 1977.

[§]For an informative article on unnatural footwear and other perversions, see "The Fashionable Body," *Horizon*, Vol. XIII, No. 4, Autumn, 1971.

[||]Various styles of Kung-Fu slippers are available from Asian World of Martial Arts (AWMA), 11601 Caroline Road, Philadelphia, PA 19154-2177, 1-800-345-2962, www.awma.com.

develop the idea next that these additions are undesirable. In my book on T'ai Chi,* I have treated additional aspects of feet and footwear and have described Native American footwear, which I believe to be the most natural.

SOLES ON SHOES

The first footwear probably consisted of an animal skin wrapped around the foot. Later, when skills of knotting, cutting, needle making, and sewing developed, it was possible to make shoes out of sections of leather that were stitched together. Then it was possible to add a protective sole made of stronger, thicker hide. Very recently, the advances in glues and synthetic sole materials have made it possible to have a large variety of materials for soles for many different uses.

For shoes I make myself, my preference is for a lightweight, soft, springy foam sole material called "cloud." The thickness of sole material is measured in "irons," one iron equaling one forty-eighth of an inch. I find that 18-iron (3/8in.) cloud is best for the shoes I make.†

Shoe soles should have enough thickness to cushion the feet, but unnecessary thickness produces leverage that makes it easy to twist and sprain an ankle or knee. At present, inordinately thick soles are in style. Observe how clumsily people walk when wearing shoes with these soles.

HEELS ON SHOES

The origin of heels on footwear is believed to date back to the Dark Ages. During that period, plumbing was nonexistent, and streets were strewn with human and animal excrement. Heels were a way of lifting the feet as high as possible above the ground. After their utilitarian function diminished, heels became an accepted style, possibly because they make the legs appear longer and seemingly more elegant.

Unfortunately, heels on shoes, even low ones, have a number of undesirable effects. Heels prevent you from experiencing the optimal length of your stride, place extra pressure on the front of the foot (see the section about bunions in Chapter 10), foreshorten the Achilles' tendon, and lead to incorrect alignment of the vertebrae of the lumbar spine. Another problem with heels is that they create leverage that can make the difference between getting an injury from improper alignment and not.

*Robert Chuckrow, *The Tai Chi Book*, YMAA Publication Center, Boston MA, 1998, pp. 130–134.

†This material is available from A & B Leather and Shoe Findings Co., Inc., 769 10th Avenue, New York, NY 10019.

As mentioned in Chapter 3, heels lift the back of the legs, causing the body to tilt forward. To compensate, the top of the body must then lean backward, thus accentuating the lumbar curve of the spine ("sway-back").

INSOLES

In the early days of making my own footwear, one of my students pointed out to me that my shoes had no cushioning other than the rubber sole. He suggested fleece-covered, foam insoles, which are available in many variety stores. Even though my feet are size eight, their large EEEEE width required that I buy the largest size, 13, and cut them down to length. I found that these insoles were indispensable and made it feel as though I were walking on clouds. Of course, I made the next pair of shoes a bit larger to accommodate the extra bulk of the insoles.

I finally located the manufacturer of the insoles and convinced the sales department to sell me a roll of hundreds of square feet of the uncut material, which I have continued to use to date.

It is a good idea to replace insoles every few weeks as they collect bacteria and become compressed with use.

ORTHOTICS

Whereas some orthotics may have a valid function, they do not get to the root of a problem that can be easily remedied by natural means. A number of my T'ai-Chi students have been able to get along without orthotics after being taught correct alignment of their feet and practicing it for a week or so.

People who flatten their arches or have other undesirable habits of walking usually take no responsibility in the matter. They characterize the poor alignment of their feet by saying "My feet are flat," as though their feet were not under their conscious control. They change their view only when shown that, with a little effort, they can attain perfect alignment. Chapter 3 contains a detailed treatment of how to achieve optimal alignment of the feet without using artificial means.

LEATHER, CLOTH, OR PLASTIC SHOES?

I studied meditation with the late Alice Holtman for a number of years. She was the vice president of the North American Vegetarian Society. One day I asked her why she, a strict ethical vegetarian, wore leather shoes. She replied, "I have tried wearing plastic shoes, but they are much too uncomfortable. At present, leather is a by-product of the meat industry. Animals are bred primarily for food, not for leather. The same number of cows would be slaughtered even if no one bought leather shoes. I avoid using leather in all other items, but giving up wearing leather shoes would be too much of a sacrifice."

Plastic is being increasingly used for making shoes. Plastic shoes tear easily and tend not to breathe. Air is very important for feet, which require oxygen, ventilation, and evaporation of perspiration.

Whereas cloth affords minimal protection, it is a very comfortable material for footwear. Cloth allows air to penetrate to the feet, bringing oxygen and helping perspiration to evaporate. Cloth-topped Kung-Fu slippers, previously mentioned, are made with three types of soles: rubber, plastic, or cloth.

SHOELACES OR VELCRO?

There is a reluctance to replace the time-tested way of doing things with some newfangled way. So, it was with much caution that I started using Velcro fastenings in the footwear I make. Velcro has an advantage over shoelaces in speed of fastening and releasing. Undoing an unwanted knot in a shoelace requires the right length fingernails, supernormal vision, and a lot of dexterity. Also, Velcro tends to stay put much more than do shoelaces. Of course, shoelaces will become untied if an incorrect knot is used (see next section). Tying the correct knot, a square knot is no guarantee. That knot relies on tension being applied continuously, which is not always the case.

Velcro compares in importance with other major historical advances such as fire, the wheel, and the back-scratcher.*

TYING SHOELACES

Many people whose shoelaces frequently become untied may simply be tying the wrong knot. The two basic knots, the granny bow and the square-knot bow, are very similar (see Figs. 9-1and 9-2 for the difference between a granny knot and a square knot and Fig. 9-3 for directions for tying a proper bow). The granny becomes very quickly untied, whereas the square knot can stay tied much longer. The square knot is tied right over left and then left over right, whereas the granny is tied right over left and then right over left again. Because most people do

*Just kidding!

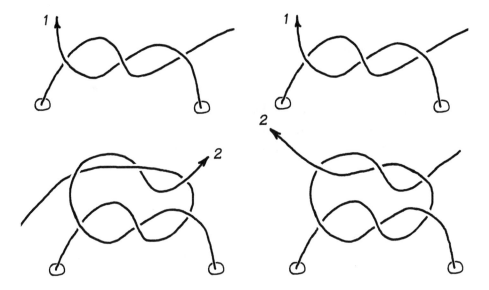

Fig. 9-1. *Square knot.(1) right over left and through, (2) left over right and through. The square knot should only be used for applications for which the knot is always under tension.*

Fig. 9-2. *Granny knot. (1) right over left and through, (2) right over left and through.*

not distinguish between these two knots, about half of the people in any group will have tied their shoelaces incorrectly.

When tied correctly, the bow will lie perpendicular to the axis of the foot, that is, from one side of the ankle to the other. When tied incorrectly, the bow will lie parallel to the axis of the foot, that is, from ankle to middle toe.

If you find that you are one of the 50 percent who tie their shoes incorrectly, simply reverse the first overhand knot, but tie the next part in the usual manner. This change should do the trick.

For extra holding strength with no loss in ease of untying your shoelaces by pulling opposite free ends, you can double the winding in step (3) of Fig. 9-3. A more-secure bow is shown in Fig. 9-4. Numerous ways of tying bows on shoes and lacing them—plus about four-thousand other knots—are given by Ashley* in his impressive treatise.

*Clifford W. Ashley, *The Ashley Book of Knots*, Doubleday & Company, Garden City, NY, 1944, pp. 221 and 331.

SOCKS

In warm weather, cotton socks with perhaps a small amount of nylon reinforcing are the best. In cold weather, heavy-duty merino wool socks, worn over cotton socks, are very warm. Campmor, Inc.* is a good source for a variety of merino wool socks and a whole host of other clothing and camping items.

LOOSE CLOTHING

In the early 1970s, skin-tight clothing came into style. About then, I had just begun studying T'ai Chi and felt the need for looser, less restrictive clothing. I remember going into a clothing store and finding that pants were so narrow at the bottoms that I could not get them over my EEEEE-wide feet. I also remember asking the salesperson if wider pants were available. His annoying response, "This is the way they're wearing them," prompted me to make my own pants. I took a pair of flannel pajama bottoms, added a drawstring of 1/2-inch twill tape, sewed up the fly, and dyed them black. I started wearing these pants only for prac-

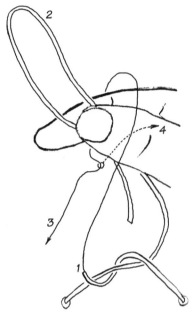

Fig. 9-3. *Basic shoelace bow. (1) Weave the right shoelace over and under the left one. (2) Pinch the right shoelace between the thumb and forefinger of your right hand. At the same time, using the thumb of your left hand as a hook, form a loop of the right shoelace. Continue to pinch the base of the loop between thumb and forefinger of your right hand. (3) With your left hand, wind the free end of the shoelace around your right thumb. (4) Hold the loop with your left hand. At the same time, using the forefinger of your right hand, pull the standing part of the right shoelace through the shoelace wound over your right thumb and forefinger to form a second loop. The knot is formed by pulling loops 2 and 4 apart. Tension must be maintained throughout the whole process.*

ticing T'ai Chi but ended up wearing them as regular pants in public.

Eventually, I opened all the seams of one pair and created a pattern for pants that I make and wear to this day. I have found that the most comfortable material is 100% cotton corduroy. The addition of polyester strengthens the material and makes it more durable but less comfortable to wear. The height of the crotch is critical; a low crotch will

*Campmor, Inc., PO Box 700, Saddle River, NJ 07458, 1-800-226-7667, www.campmor.com.

chafe your thighs and a high crotch will restrict your movements.

SUSPENDERS

About twenty years ago, one of my physics students, David Franklin, noticed that I frequently needed to adjust the height of my drawstring pants. He suggested that I try wearing suspenders, and I have continued wearing them to this day. I find that the freedom of abdominal motion during breathing is very important.

When the elastic becomes weak, it is easy to replace. In my opinion, elastic bought from a fabric store is usually of a higher quality than that of the original suspenders.

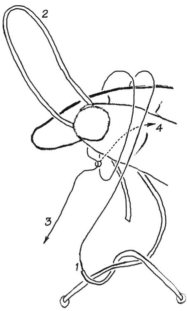

Fig. 9-4. More-secure shoelace bow. Same as in Fig. 9–3 except that a double winding is formed in step (3).

WARM CLOTHING

Those who are experienced in outdoor activities seem to agree that wool and goose down are preferable to "man-made" fibers. These natural materials breathe, allowing perspiration to evaporate and oxygen to penetrate. Wool retains its thermal properties even when wet.

CHAPTER 10

Walking Safely

AUTOMOBILES

As an experienced driver, I am often amazed at how many people wear dark clothing at night and seem unaware of how difficult it is to see them. They apparently think that if they can see you, you can see them—the inverse of the ostrich principle. When walking at night—or at any time, for that matter—you should always assume that drivers do not see you. When road conditions permit, walk on the side of the road facing oncoming traffic so you can see cars coming and move safely out of their way if necessary.

A compact, bright-red, clip-on flashing safety light is available in stores selling sports equipment. Such lights are typically powered by two AA cells and can be seen half a mile away. Various reflective stripes and "blaze-orange" safety vests are also readily available.

POLLUTION

When you walk on a road, keep in mind that car and truck exhaust fumes contain carbon monoxide and a host of other pollutants. Try to find a place to walk where traffic is sparse, or walk during a low-volume part of the day. The best place to walk is near dense vegetation, which emits large quantities of oxygen, especially in the early morning.

When I lived in Brooklyn, I regularly rode my bicycle in Prospect Park on Saturdays when it was closed to traffic. One Saturday, I started to feel faint and made my way home. A friend with whom I was riding stayed behind. When I got home, I noticed a strong chemical odor coming from my clothes. On the radio I heard that the pollution levels were characterized as "dangerous." I phoned my friend, who by now was also home. He also noticed the odor and was now feeling sick. The next day, he developed a serious cough, which continued for a few weeks.

Whereas I had no proof that our symptoms had resulted from air pollution, I began to be much more aware of the correlation between the degree of pollution and how I felt. From then on, I abstained from running or bicycling on days when the air pollution was high (as observed personally or from weather advisories).

SUNBURN

In recent years it has been common for people to use sunscreen preparations. However, these preparations may be harmful. Whereas a sunscreen protects against the rays that cause burning, it may not protect against the rays that cause cancer. Or, the sunscreen may be itself harmful. The best course is to realize that the skin builds up its own natural protection to the harmful effects of the sun through the production of the dark pigment, melanin. The presence of melanin is commonly called a *suntan*.

Each genetic type has a different capacity to produce melanin. People with blond or red hair or with blue eyes are much more susceptible to the sun than those with dark hair. Of course, dark-skinned people whose ancestors originated in tropical areas of the world have the greatest capacity to withstand the sun.

When exposure to the sun is reduced, the melanin becomes absorbed. This adaptation makes sense because sunlight is necessary, and too much melanin would excessively block vital sunlight. Thus, during winter, when exposure to the sun is greatly reduced, protection diminishes. The problem arises when there is a sudden rather than gradual increase in exposure. Upon the return of warm weather, it is common for those who have lost most of their protection against strong sunlight to suddenly expose themselves to hours of intense sunlight on the first clear, bright day. They receive not only direct sunlight but also the ultraviolet light reflected by the sky. The amount of exposure is then many times the optimal amount, and, of course, damage occurs.

It should be understood that the effect on melanin production in response to an increased exposure to the sun takes about two weeks to develop. With this fact in mind, you should become attuned to your individual degree of vulnerability to the sun, and slowly work up to the point where full exposure is safe.

Excessive exposure is evidenced by reddening the next day or by eventual blistering and loss of one or more layers of the skin. Once the skin has been overexposed to sunlight, damage of a serious nature has occurred. At that point, you should *get no further exposure until the skin has completely healed.* Then, buildup very slowly to give the new skin ample opportunity to become protected.

The use of soap removes natural oils from the skin that protect it from the harmful effects of sunlight. It is also likely that a dietary deficiency of undamaged* fats rich in essential fatty acids lowers the protective ability of the skin. Raw flax seeds, pumpkin seeds, and walnuts are rich in the essential fatty acids. Eating them produces a healthy, silky, glowing skin.

Excessive exposure to sunlight produces free-radical damage within the living cells below the surface of the skin. This damage is somewhat offset by antioxidants such as vitamin E. If you anticipate that you may be overexposed to the sun, try taking 1,000 i.u. (international units) of vitamin E beforehand. This precaution is said to vastly reduce susceptibility to sunburn.[†] My experience has borne out this protective effect.

POISON IVY

Poison ivy is a climbing plant with sets of three leaves. Each leaf has serrated edges (see Fig. 10-1). If you think that your skin has been exposed to the leaves or stems, try to wash the affected areas thoroughly with a tincture of green soap or any other strong soap. If you do end up with poison ivy, which consists of a rash and/or blisters, you may achieve immediate and possibly permanent relief by heating the area with a hair dryer for about ten seconds. Get the area as hot as possible without burning yourself. My conjecture is that this remedy works because the heat breaks down the substances that cause the extreme itching.

If you want to eliminate poison ivy plants, do not think that you can put on rubber gloves and pull them out. Unless you cover your entire body, the vapor released will reach exposed parts of your skin such as your face. Instead of pulling poison ivy out, use a commercial herbicide specifically for it. A tiny amount of this spray applied to each

---

*Fats—especially polyunsaturated ones—are highly susceptible to free-radical production from heat, light, and oxygen. For that reason, vegetable oils are unsuitable for cooking. Partially hydrogenated vegetable oil is liquid oil that has been purposely damaged to achieve a consistency resembling that of butter or lard. For a more complete discussion on the beneficial and harmful aspects of dietary fats, see Chuckrow, *The Intelligent Dieter's Guide*, Rising Mist Publication, Briarcliff Manor, P.O. Box 50, NY 10510, 1997, pp 10-14.

[†]Gary Price Todd, M.D., *Nutrition, Health, & Disease*, Whitford Press, West Chester, PA, 1985, p.135.

intersection of three leaves will cause the plant to wither and die in a few days.

LIGHTNING

More people are struck by lightning per year than you might imagine. It is important to know what to do when walking outdoors during a thunderstorm. Many people seek shelter under a tree when it starts to rain. Unfortunately,

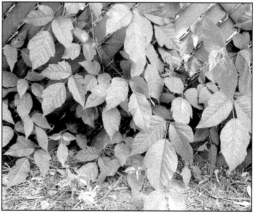

Fig. 10-1. *Poison ivy. Note the distinctive groups of three leaves with serrated edges.*

the tree may be struck by lightning, which produces two problems: (1) The tree or part of it may fall on you, and (2) the electrical effect of being that close to a lightning strike can be harmful.

Being hit by lightning need not be fatal. People in top physical condition can survive being hit by lightning much better than people who are weak or in poor health. Some people have been hit more than once.

When lightning strikes, the safest place to be is in an automobile (not a convertible)—but not if the car is parked under a tree, which can fall on the car if the tree is hit. The reason the car is the safest place is not, as many think, because the tires are made of rubber! When lightning strikes a car, huge sparks jump from the body of the car to the ground, so any possible insulation provided by the tires is meaningless. A car is safe because you are almost completely enclosed by metal when inside it. Over two-hundred years ago, Michael Faraday demonstrated by means of his "ice-pail experiment" that there can be no electrical effects inside a cavity in a conductor—no matter what happens outside.

If you lack a car and are in an open area, it may be best to lie down flat on the ground—especially if you feel the electricity on your skin or traveling through your head to your feet. Of course, you may get drenched and muddy, but standing involves a serious risk.

One common misconception is that lightning never strikes twice in the same spot. The towers on the top of the Empire State Building are frequently hit by lightning, and there are quite a few photographs documenting these repeated hits.

THE FOLLOWING PERSONAL LIGHTNING SAFETY TIPS ARE OFFERED BY THE NATIONAL LIGHTNING SAFETY INSTITUTE:

1. Plan in advance your evacuation and safety measures. When you first see lightning or hear thunder, activate your emergency plan. Now is the time to go to a building or a vehicle. Lightning often precedes rain, so don't wait for the rain to begin before suspending activities.

2. If outdoors, avoid water. Avoid the high ground. Avoid open spaces. Avoid all metal objects including electric wires, fences, machinery, motors, power tools, etc. Unsafe places include underneath canopies, small picnic or rain shelters, or near trees. Where possible, find shelter in a substantial building or in a fully enclosed metal vehicle such as a car, truck or a van with the windows completely shut. If lightning is striking nearby when you are outside, you should:

   a) Crouch down. Put feet together. Place hands over ears to minimize hearing damage from thunder.

   b) Avoid proximity (minimum of 15 ft) to other people.

3. If indoors, avoid water. Stay away from doors and windows. Do not use the telephone. Take off head sets. Turn off, unplug, and stay away from appliances, computers, power tools, & TV sets. Lightning may strike exterior electric and phone lines, inducing shocks to inside equipment.

4. Suspend activities for 30 minutes after the last observed lightning or thunder.

5. Injured people do not carry an electrical charge and can be handled safely. Apply First Aid procedures to a lightning victim if you are qualified to do so. Call 911 or send for help immediately. Know your emergency telephone numbers.

From the National Lightning Safety Institute, 891 N. Hoover Ave.,
Louisville, CO 80027 (lightning safety.com)

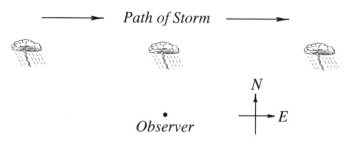

Fig. 10-2. *Thunderstorm to north of observer, moving eastward. Distance of storm from observer decreases and then increases.*

It is useful to know how to tell how far you are from a lightning strike. Because sound travels about 1,000 feet per second in air and one mile is 5,280 feet, thunder will be delayed by about five seconds for each mile the lightning strike is distant. You can sometimes monitor the advance or retreat of a storm by noting the increase or decrease in the delay. For example, a delay that first increases and then decreases indicates that you are not in the path of the storm and that the storm is now receding (see Fig. 10-2).

DEHYDRATION

Consumption of the proper amount of water has become an issue that has been widely publicized in recent years. Drinking too much water is not a good idea because it tends to leach out vital nutrients and places a strain on the kidneys to remove the excess. On the other hand, the ill effects of dehydration are much more serious, so it is better to err on the side of too much water. The main symptoms of dehydration are sluggishness of body and mind ("brain fog").

In an extremely critical situation, when you are in danger of dying of thirst and no water is available, it may save your life to drink your own urine. The *US Army Survival Manual*,* which is a reprint of the Department of Army Field Manual FM 21-76, includes an excellent chapter on water procurement plus a wealth of other information.

TICKS

Various species of ticks live in many parts of the United States, and some can transmit serious diseases. Dog ticks, which tend to be large, can carry Rocky Mountain Spotted Fever. So-called "deer ticks," which are very small, can carry Lyme disease. The larval stages of deer ticks

US Army Field Manual, Dorset Press, New York, 1991, Ch. 5.

grow on the white-footed mouse, and the adult ticks tend to live on deer and sometimes other mammals.

I have never, to my knowledge, experienced a tick bite, but recently my dog did. She had been lying in the grass, and there was a large dog tick embedded in the inside of her ear. I remembered the admonition not to pull out the tick and leave its mouth parts. After I tried to dislodge the tick various ways, it became apparent that it was not going to be pulled off easily.

Next, I looked up "ticks" in my copy of *Merck's Manual*,* a medical reference book that every household should have. Merck's suggested swabbing the area with alcohol, grabbing the *head* of the engorged tick with tweezers, and applying gradual traction until the tick is dislodged. After a few tries, I managed to pull it off along with a small part of my dog's ear in its mandibles. Surprisingly, my dog seemed to realize that I was trying to help her and was totally cooperative all through the ordeal.

After being outdoors for a period of time during warmer months, it is a good idea to carefully inspect your legs and other exposed parts of your body. Serrated-tipped tweezers are the best kind to use for tick removal.

Mosquitoes

When a mosquito bites, it injects a digestive enzyme that breaks down your tissues, releasing your blood. The mosquito then extracts the blood. If disturbed before finishing its meal, the mosquito flies away, leaving the injected enzyme, which causes the itching characteristic of a mosquito bite. Supposedly, if a mosquito is allowed to finish its meal, it draws back all of the enzyme that, otherwise, would cause itching.

Several summers ago, I was sitting quietly when, suddenly, a mosquito landed on my thigh just below my shorts. As a scientific experiment, I decided to permit the mosquito to feed freely. I watched the abdomen of the mosquito become increasingly large for a period of time; the insect was so quiet that I began to think it was dead or asleep. Finally, when its abdomen had grown to enormous proportions, the mosquito suddenly zoomed off.

Using ink, I drew a circle around the site, which itched slightly. The next day, there was no itching or redness. In fact, without the identifying circle I had drawn, there was no way of knowing where the bite was.

*The Merck *Manual of Diagnosis and Therapy*, Published by Merck Research Laboratories, Rahway, NJ, 16th Edition, 1992, pp. 174–5.

THORNS

Having a thorn embedded in your finger can be very uncomfortable. Recently, while asleep, I became aware of severe itching that seemed to radiate from my hand, all the way up my arm, and then into my chest. When I awoke, I examined my hand and saw what appeared to be a small raised area. I assumed that I must have touched poison ivy while picking berries the day before. I applied the hair-dryer treatment for poison ivy just described and got complete relief. That evening, I noticed that there appeared to be a dark spot under the raised area. It turned out to be a thorn from a berry bush.

The way I like to remove a thorn (or splinter) is to use a sail needle. Such a needle has a long, tapered, very sharp, triangular point. I always carry one of these needles embedded in a business card. Another useful item is a small magnifying glass—preferably one that can be used hands-free.

WALKING SURFACES

Living in a relatively rural area, I frequently see people walking, or worse, running on concrete or macadam instead of adjacent grass or earth. In terms of the impact to your body and the effect on your feet, there is an important difference between a natural surface and a surface that has no give. When an action is repeated many times in succession, as in walking or running, seemingly small factors become quite important. There is a Chinese saying, "Constant grinding can turn an iron bar into a needle."

An advantage of walking on natural ground instead of pavement is that small variations in contour have the effect of massaging your feet. Moreover, a natural surface requires using your eyes to see, your body to feel, and your brain to process in order to accommodate your footing and movements to constantly changing conditions.

DOGS

Dogs are usually polite because they know that they are living in a human world in a dependent mode. However, dogs, like humans, are affected by past experiences, low blood sugar, and the phases of the moon. The presence of children brings out dogs' protective instincts and makes them more likely to bite.

When I was in my late teens, I had a job as a door-to-door salesperson for a few summers. Being outdoors in unfamiliar neighborhoods provided an opportunity for me to observe a variety of ways that dogs react to strangers. Many dogs just want to make friends, and their barking is friendly. Dogs also read the expression on your face to determine whether or not you are there as a friend. Smiling softly will have a very beneficial effect.

Angry dogs are usually cowards, and some would rather bite you from behind. They will think twice about coming near you when they see that you are observant and are carrying an object they think can be used to hurt them. I found that holding a clipboard in an extended fashion noticeably deterred dogs from approaching me.

In some areas, dogs roam in packs. Usually they are in a good mood because they like running around with each other. However, it is very important to be cautious.

Unless you are already friends with a dog, resist the impulse to pet it, even when the owner says, "my dog doesn't bite." Every dog that ever bit someone did it a first time.

FLEAS

Fleas live in the hair of animals and feed on their blood. Fleas apparently become bored with living in the same abode and eating the same food. They like variety. As a human, you are a handy provider of temporary room, board, and transportation until a suitable cat or dog appears.

Fleas carry diseases that they transmit to their host. Bubonic plague was transmitted by fleas from rats to humans and still sparsely exists the world over. Fleas also transmit certain parasitic diseases. Fleas live for years and can go for many months without a meal.

Years ago, two squirrels took up residence in my attic. I dispossessed them using a "Havahart" trap and a lot of ingenuity. Unfortunately, their fleas remained. When I approached the area where the squirrels had been, about half a dozen fleas immediately jumped on my legs. After killing the fleas that were feeding on me, I avoided the attic during the whole winter into spring. When I again ventured into the attic, I saw fleas feebly trying to jump. They were still alive! By the end of spring, they were virtually dead except for slight occasional movements of their feet.

Fleas can also withstand extreme pressure. Squeezing one between thumb and forefinger will have little effect. To kill a flea, you need to cut it in half with the edge of your thumbnail.

Because they are tough, fleas living on you like to bite you while ensconced under the elastic of your underwear or socks or in the crease where your buttocks join with your legs. Their bites are typically in groups of two or three and itch intensely. Fleas spend time around their host's bed and can be eliminated by cleaning that area with a vacuum cleaner whose bag contains a few mothballs. *National Geographic** has a fascinating, comprehensive, and beautifully illustrated article on fleas.

FLIES

One or more flies buzzing around your head can be quite annoying. Some of them (deer flies) bite painfully and may even spread disease. I have found that the way to get rid of a circling fly is to tilt your head backward, so your eyes point upward. Then try to clap the fly with your hands. Even if you miss, the fly will realize that it is in danger and look for a different host.

FOREIGN OBJECT IN EYE

A tiny piece of dirt in your eye is not only uncomfortable but can lead to a serious problem. Usually, simply closing the affected eye for a few minutes will allow tears to float the debris out. If the tears do not do the job, it is a good idea to locate the dirt. If the dirt is on the inside of the lower lid, it can be carefully swept out with a cotton swab. If the dirt is embedded in the cornea (the clear region) for more than a few hours, it probably is a good idea to enlist the services of a professional. Debris in the cornea can move inward, and once it does, removal is essentially impossible.

STRANGERS

It is disconcerting to be approached by a stranger when walking alone in an isolated area. Whereas most such situations are innocuous, the response to any negative intuitive feeling on your part should be to run away. Do not worry about offending a stranger by your quick departure!

---

*N. Duplaix., "Fleas, the Lethal Leapers," *National Geographic*, Vol. 173, No. 5, May 1988, pp. 671–694.

SELF-PROTECTION TOOLS

It is desirable to carry a walking stick or martial arts hanbo,*† which is a 36-inch-long hardwood staff 1 inch in diameter. A stick can be carried hanging vertically in a neutral position, resting against the web between the thumb and forefinger of the hand ("tiger's mouth"), with the arm and hand hanging naturally by the side. This carrying position can easily change to other grasps, such as carrying the stick in a closed fist as the other end of the hanbo arcs forward or to the side. In the neutral hand position, the stick can arc backward to be concealed behind the arm or easily be transferred to the other hand, in the opposite grip. A stick can be used for striking and as an extension of your arm for snaking movements to achieve joint locks on your attacker.

Keys can be effectively used for self-defense at short range. Place the key ring in the palm of one hand, with three keys protruding outward, each between two fingers. Orient the serrations so they are toward the tips of the fingers. The keys become like claws and can be used in a slashing manner.

A nylon ("unbreakable") comb can be held with the wider end in the palm and the narrower end naturally extending between the thumb and forefinger. The comb can be used for slashing with the tines or striking with the end.

Knives of all types are widely available and have many uses other than protection in the event of an attack by a dog or person. In some instances, knives can be as dangerous as firearms, and there are many laws restricting the length, ways of opening, and ways of carrying knives. It is very important that you ascertain what lengths and types the local ordinances permit and stay within the law.

It is always important that you carry any self-protection tools in a non-threatening manner. Otherwise, the probability of needing to use the tool is increased. Also, a tool is most effective when it surprises the attacker and, therefore, reduces his ability to take the tool into consideration.

Many people feel that a pistol is the most desirable self-protection tool. Pistols are very highly regulated by the government, and owning a

*In Japanese, *hanbo* means half bo. The bo is a six-foot staff that was widely used for self protection in Japan's feudal days.

†The following is an excellent and comprehensive book of self-defense techniques using a stick: Masaaki Hatsumi and Quinton Chambers, *Stick Fighting*, Kodansha International Ltd., New York, 1981, ISBN 0-97011-475-1.

pistol requires a federal background check and a waiting period. The more rural the area, the more lax the local laws and the easier and more quickly you can obtain a "carry permit." In most cities, it is essentially impossible to get an unrestricted permit that allows carrying a pistol. In some localities, it is even hard to get a permit that allows you to carry the pistol to a target range or to an area where hunting is permitted.

Owning a firearm of any type is very dangerous and a bad idea unless (a) the firearm and the ammunition are properly stored, (b) you and others in your family are trained in firearm safety, and (c) you become fully knowledgeable about the laws governing the use of deadly force. Of course, everyone—martial artist, firearm owner, and humble, unarmed, private citizen—should know these important laws, which vary from state to state. Keep in mind that any object can be legally considered a weapon when used to harm someone other than for legal self-defense.*

First-Aid Kit

A few small, carefully chosen items can be indispensable when away from home. I usually take along a kit consisting of a sail needle (with a tapered, very sharp triangular point), a small magnifying glass, mirror, assorted adhesive bandage strips, a roll of clear surgical tape, a small pair of surgical tweezers, toothpicks, dental floss or tape, assorted safety pins, a sewing needle and thread, a single-edged razor blade (safely wrapped), a few tissues neatly folded and placed in a sealable plastic bag, a bunch of cotton swabs, and a half-ounce bottle of dit da jow (described in Chapter 11 entitled *Foot, Ankle, Leg, and Knee Problems*).

Safety pins provide a quick, temporary repair for torn clothing or a substitute for lost, buttons. Dental floss can also be used as strong string for tying things.

Flashlight

Recently, I was walking in darkness along a brick path from someone's house to an asphalt-paved driveway where my car had been parked earlier, during daylight. The two other people walking with me were finding it difficult to see, so I decided to go ahead to my car to get a large flashlight. I actually had a small flashlight in my shoulder bag but did not want to look for it in the dark. I went ahead, not realizing that there was a series of three steps, each separated by about a stride of

---

*A good starting book is Karl J. Duff, *Martial Arts & the Law*, Ohara Publications, Inc., Burbank, CA, 1985.

horizontal path. I missed the first step, and foolishly tried to catch my balance, only to miss the next step. By the time I missed the third step, I was moving with considerable momentum and found myself flying forward in the darkness.

I landed on the asphalt driveway on my hands, hitting my knees. At first, I thought that I had fractured one of my kneecaps because the pain was so intense. After a few minutes of sending ch'i to the area, the pain was almost gone. I ended up with only a small scrape on my left knee and right palm. When I got home, I applied some dit da jow to my knee and, by then, knew that the injury was innocuous. The next day I was able to attain the "Downward Single Whip" posture of the T'ai-Chi form without any problem.

Whereas such mishaps are embarrassing and humbling, they provide valuable insights. I have since certainly made up my mind to take whatever time necessary to retrieve my small flashlight whenever a need for it is even suggested. Also, I realize that I was too confident in my abilities. However, even though it was totally dark and I had no way of *thinking* how to react, my body knew how to protect itself. The fact that my triceps were sore the next day indicated that I had applied a large supporting force with my hands as I received the ground. The fact that I did not injure my fingers or wrists meant that I had regulated the pressure to be below a harmful level and had not stiffened my fingers, wrists, or arms. I also confirmed my ability to accelerate the healing process using ch'i and herbs.

Although I had reacted reasonably well, in retrospect, it would have been better to have dropped to the ground immediately instead of trying to regain my balance. Of course, I would not have fallen at all had I exercised more caution in walking in the dark. Had I utilized my small flashlight, I would not have even needed to walk in the dark.

Many inexpensive, dependable, light-weight, and compact flashlights are available by mail-order or in sporting-goods stores. Various small but very bright flashlights using one or two AA or AAA alkaline batteries are also available for about $10 each. Flashlights using light-emitting diodes (LEDs) are extremely small (about the size of a quarter) and use one or two 3-volt lithium batteries, each about the size and shape of a penny (see Fig. 10-3). They come in various colors of light—red, blue, green, yellow, and white, listed here in order of increasing delay of recovering night vision after your eyes are exposed to their light. Most LED flashlights cost about $10–$20 and weigh only a fraction of an ounce with batteries. The LED bulbs emit less light than their incandescent counterparts but are much more energy-efficient and can "burn" for 100,000+ hours (over 11 years) without failure.

The advantage of a small flashlight is its light weight, which allows it to be carried on a key ring or, for ready use, on a lanyard around your neck.

Headlamps are also available for extended, comfortable, hands-free use at night. At least two designs of headlamps incorporate an array of three LEDs, ample to illuminate a path. Headlamps range in price from about $10 to $66.

IDENTIFICATION CARD

It is wise to carry an identification card at all times and essential when walking in a remote region. Include your name, address, phone number, emergency phone number, physician's name and phone number, allergies to medicines, and any health conditions that might need to be known in case you become hospitalized for some reason.

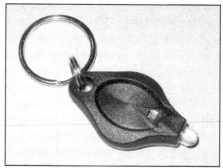

Fig. 10-3. *An LED key-chain flashlight. The design shown incorporates an on/off switch for continuous lighting as well as a momentary squeeze switch.*

SENSITIVITY TO DANGER

A few years ago, one of my T'ai-Chi students told me that while she was in a restaurant, a strange feeling came over her that someone was going to steal her purse. She was embarrassed to exhibit mistrust of others nearby and disregarded her intuition. Her purse was stolen shortly afterwards.

My response to her was that intuition should always be listened to and heeded. If intuition is disregarded, it becomes stunted; if taken seriously, it becomes strengthened and increasingly reliable.

There is a famous story of a pupil of a highly accomplished master.* While the master was in the garden absorbed in picking and arranging flowers, the pupil had the thought that he could launch a surprise

*Oscar Ratti and Adele Westbrook, *Secrets of the Samurai,* Charles E. Tuttle Company, Inc., Rutland, VT, 1973, p. 392.

attack on the seemingly preoccupied master. Immediately, the master began to scan the horizon, waiting for an impending attack. For days, the master was in an evident state of readiness. Finally, the pupil confessed what had happened, whereupon the master relaxed.

When intention to do harm is present, the air seems to crackle with a negative energy the Ninja calls *sakki*, "the intent of the killer."* Those sensitive to sakki experience an urgent feeling of danger. It is when we suppress this valuable intuition that we get into trouble.

RUNNING AWAY FROM DANGER

Most martial arts training emphasizes standing your ground and fighting. Except for certain situations, running away is usually the most desirable alternative. Of course, running away may not be feasible if we need to protect another person.

Most of us have been taught from an early age not to run away but face whatever we are afraid of. In school, we take a test whether we are prepared or not. If we receive a letter requiring us to do jury duty, we respond responsibly. However, our ancestors a hundred-thousand years ago dealt with danger by running away, just as wild animals do. There are times when we need to listen to and obey our urge to flee.

---

*For a discussion of sakki, see Stephen K. Hayes, *The Ninja and their Secret Fighting Art*, Charles E. Tuttle Company, Inc., Rutland VT, 1981, pp. 144–8.

CHAPTER 11

Foot, Ankle, Leg, and Knee Problems

ALIGNMENT

Improper alignment is at the root of most foot, ankle, and knee problems. Chronic injury can result from the repetitive action of walking with joints off center, under stress. Moreover, incorrect alignment greatly increases the probability of an acute trauma.

You should attempt to correct the alignment of your feet, ankles and knees by (a) practicing the exercises pertaining to the centers of the feet (outlined in Chapter 3) and (b) manifesting these concepts in your spontaneous movements.

BUNIONS

A bunion is "an inflammatory swelling of the bursa over the metatarsophalangeal joint of the big toe."* The formation of bunions is evidently a consequence of chronic excess harmful pressure on the first metatarsal (base of the big toe). The excess pressure can be caused by a combination of factors. Over the years that I have been teaching T'ai Chi and observing people's feet, their deformities, and improper usage, I have noticed that women have bunions much more often than men. Moreover, women who wear high-heeled shoes have the most severe cases. Such shoes place an inordinate pressure on the ball of the foot. Even when "flat" footwear is worn, the habitual placement of pressure on the ball of the foot continues to take its toll. Of course, shoes that are pointed in front squeeze the big toe inward, further increasing the pressure on the first metatarsal.

Another factor is habitually caving in the arch, which places even more pressure on and rubbing of the first metatarsal (see "Fallen Arches," next section).

Recovery from bunions is slow, and can occur only when both the

*Stedman's Medical Dictionary, The Williams &Wilkinson Co., Baltimore, MD, 1966.

habits of usage and the offending footwear are eliminated. Just as the bone absorbed extra calcium and grew larger, the calcium build-up can be eventually absorbed, with the consequent reduction in size of the bunions.

The exercises described in Chapter 3 will be found to be valuable in reeducating patterns of foot usage.

FALLEN ARCHES

"I have fallen arches" is an expression that conveys a lack of responsibility in the matter. If you walked around with your head tilted 45 degrees to one side, your friends would wonder why you would do such a thing. Characterizing your head as having fallen to one side would not be accepted as a valid reason, and people would expect you to remedy the situation by lifting your head. However, responsibility is not expected when it comes to the lowest part of the body although, in almost all cases, fallen arches are self-inflicted. The problem arises when the center of the weight distribution on the sole of the foot is not over the center of the foot but shifted inward. Fallen arches are usually eliminated in a short time by conscientiously practicing finding the centers of the feet and centering the weight distribution there (see the section titled "Finding the Centers of the Feet" in Chapter 3).

INGROWN TOENAILS

Overly tight and stylishly pointed shoes are a main cause of ingrown toenails. The pressure on the toes causes toenails to grow into the tissues, causing pain and, sometimes, infection. People who are prone to ingrown toenails usually have toes whose outer contour parallels that of pointed shoes worn for decades. Obviously, ingrown toenails are more prevalent among women.

BLISTERS

A blister on any part of the foot is quite serious. It is best if the blister is discovered in time, that is, before it breaks. In this case, every possible precaution must be taken to prevent the blister from breaking. If the blister breaks, deeper layers of skin are exposed to bacteria and, consequently, possible infection. Apply a loose bandage with an added cotton cushion between the blister and the bandage.

CALLUSES

Calluses are formed by abrasion to the skin, which eventually dies and becomes hard and thick. Improperly fitting footwear and failure to wear socks are both factors leading to foot calluses. Once these factors are eliminated, the skin on the foot will gradually become more supple.

TENDONITIS

Tendons are fibrous bands of tissue that connect muscles to bones. When muscles contract repetitively and forcefully such as in running or in a strenuous task, the associated tendons can become inflamed and even microscopically torn. Whereas gentle movement is helpful, stressful movement exacerbates and greatly prolongs the condition. Massage, dit da jow, ch'i, and possibly magnets are of value (all of these therapies are discussed at the end of this chapter).

KNEE PAIN

Knee pain can be caused by a number of different factors. Pain just above or below the kneecap indicates a possible tendonitis. In this case, movement under stress should be avoided until recovery is complete. Regular gentle massage and application of dit da jow usually speed the recovery. Pain on one or both sides of the knee is suggestive of strained ligaments, usually caused by faulty alignment (caving the knee inward). Knee pain can also be caused by a pinched or ruptured meniscus. When the focus of the pain is the joint itself, arthritis is a possibility. Because severe damage or degeneration can be accompanied by only slight knee pain, it is wise to take any level of such pain seriously.

Vague pains in the knees, especially in teen-age boys ("growing pains") can be due to a dietary zinc deficiency. During puberty, when the sexual organs are developing, the prostate gland absorbs large amounts of zinc for its secretions. Insufficient dietary zinc can then result in a sacrifice of some of the zinc from the bones for the important evolutionary purpose of reproductive development. When my stepson was in his early teens, he developed a painful condition of the knees diagnosed as Osgood-Schlatter disease. Suspecting that zinc might be a factor, I started him on daily zinc supplements. His symptoms then subsided within one week.

A few students have come to me with severe knee pain. One student wanted to learn the T'ai-Chi form very much but was concerned that her knee pain would be prohibitive. She mentioned that a number of medical tests were done with an inconclusive outcome. I noticed that she was habitually hyperextending her knees (forcing her knees backward). After being corrected and abstaining from hyperextending her knees for a few days, she noticed a dramatic reduction of her knee pain and was able to learn the T'ai-Chi form. The first half of Chapter 3 deals with this and other alignment problems and their remedies.

Frequently, what is experienced as knee pain originates from problems above or below the knee. It is wise to thoroughly explore the regions surrounding the knee to locate the source of the pain before blaming the pain on the knee. Locating and massaging a traumatized muscle or tendon near the knee helps to sensitize you to experience pain originating at its source rather than in another spot. At least, massaging the surrounding musculature can help reduce problems originating in the knees themselves.

SWOLLEN FEET

Swollen feet can be a symptom of serious conditions such as hypothyroidism, congestive heart failure, or adrenal insufficiency. Foot massage, soaking the feet in hot water, resting the feet on a vibrating pad, and raising the feet as high as possible are of value. The only real solution is getting to the underlying cause of the condition (often an endocrine imbalance) and remedying it.

"BURNING" FEET

A burning sensation of the soles of the feet can have a number of causes, one of which is a vitamin B12 deficiency. vitamin B12 is prevalent in all animal foods such as animal flesh, milk products, and eggs. Those on a strict vegan diet (no animal products) can develop a vitamin B12 deficiency. However, meat-eaters can also develop a deficiency due to poor absorption in the intestines or because of intestinal parasites that soak up vitamin B12. You can purchase vitamin B12 in tablet form with a potency as high as 5,000 micrograms. One of these small, pink, sweet tablets is placed under the tongue, where the tablet slowly dissolves and the vitamin is absorbed directly into the blood stream.

BRUISES TO THE SHIN

When the shin bone is traumatized, it can be extremely painful and can swell to enormous proportions. Unfortunately, such injuries tend to take an inordinately long time to heal because of the reduced circulation of blood to that region.

SPRAINS

A sprain is "an injury to a joint, with a possible rupture of some of the ligaments or tendons but without dislocation or fracture."* Sprains usually result from a joint forcefully moved beyond the extreme of its range of motion. The primary way of preventing a sprain is to develop sensitivity to any displacement of your joints from the center. Then, you can feel damaging pressure and immediately yield to it.

Once a sprain occurs, the conventional treatment involves immediately packing the affected area in ice. But what if ice is not available when the sprain occurs? In this case, it is most important to experience the pain in a relaxed manner without panicking. If you know how to send ch'i to the area, do this immediately until the pain totally subsides. If you are not experienced in sending ch'i, gentle chafing of the region for about twenty minutes should substantially reduce the injury and pain. If you have dit da jow (described later in this chapter), apply it as soon as possible before chafing. The dit da jow should greatly reduce the time required for the pain to subside.

After a sprain, it is essential to allow the injury to recover completely before using the affected part in a carefree manner. If the part is re-injured before it heals, recovery will be much more difficult and lengthy.

ATHLETE'S FOOT

Untreated athlete's foot can become a systemic, chronic condition that is almost impossible to eliminate. For this reason it is important to begin treatment immediately—don't even wait one day. Over-the-counter anti-fungal creams or liquids containing the active ingredient 1% clotrimazole are inexpensive and provide a very effective cure. If you are reluctant to use the fungal preparations, you can try applying a 3% solution of hydrogen peroxide two or three times a day, which works in a mild case.

*Stedman's Medical Dictionary, The Williams & Wilkinson Co., Baltimore, 1966.

Prevention involves proper sanitation, ventilation, and hygiene of feet (see Chapter 8).

FOOT AND LEG CRAMPS

Cramps of the lower extremities most commonly occur during sleep but sometimes appear during the day. One of the prime causes of these muscle spasms is a mineral imbalance caused by too little magnesium. Many people take calcium supplements at bedtime because calcium is said to be excreted to the greatest extent during sleep. The problem is that almost no calcium supplements contain *any* magnesium. However, we need magnesium and calcium in about a one-to-two ratio. It is assumed that everyone gets enough magnesium from eating green vegetables and fresh fruits. But this assumption just does not hold these days, for many people eat fruits and green vegetables infrequently. Moreover, they eat many foods that are both low in magnesium and increase the need for it. Therefore, taking magnesium supplements is probably a good idea—especially if you take extra unbalanced calcium.

The consumption of carbonated drinks such as soda and beer is an important cause of leg or foot cramps. The dissolved carbon dioxide, which gives these drinks their "fizz," is really an acid (carbonic acid). The body is quite able to eliminate carbon dioxide, which is one of the main by-products of metabolism of food. However, when we absorb the relatively large additional amount of carbon dioxide from carbonated beverages, the blood stream becomes temporarily acidified. Calcium and magnesium are then released from the muscles to neutralize this acid. This effect is compounded during sleep, when blood circulation and the eliminative capacities of the body are reduced. The loss of calcium and magnesium from the muscles can then lead to a cramp. Cramps are more likely to occur in the lower extremities, where circulation is the least.

Just as the carbonic acid from soda or beer can be a cause of muscle spasms, so can the acid elements from food. Animal flesh, peanuts, eggs, and beans are very high in acid elements such as phosphorus, sulfur, and chlorine. It is important to balance meals containing such foods with other foods high in alkaline elements. The primary alkaline elements, calcium, and magnesium, are abundant in green, leafy vegetables.

Other causes of muscle spasms are nitrates and monosodium glutamate (MSG). Nitrates are added to processed meats to prevent them from turning brown. Nitrates are quite irritating to nerve and muscle tissue. MSG is created by combining NaCl (ordinary salt) with glutamic acid, an amino acid that naturally occurs in many foods and especially in the gluten in wheat. Because MSG occurs naturally, it is present in many foods that do not list it in the ingredients. For example, soy sauce often contains MSG that appears during the fermentation and aging process. Also, some foods have added MSG that is not listed on the label. MSG is a gastric and neurological irritant. When nerves are irritated (for any reason), they cause muscles to contract. The muscular contraction cuts off the blood supply to the nerves, which nourishes, oxygenates, and cleanses them of waste products. Thus, when the muscles unnecessarily contract, the nerves become even more irritated, causing a vicious cycle. It may take a few days for nitrates or MSG to clear out of your body, so it is best to avoid them in the first place.

Another factor in foot and leg cramps is the temperature of the lower extremities. The legs tend to be cooler than the rest of the body because of their relatively larger surface to volume ratio. During sleep, the lower temperature results in decreased circulation and, consequently, reduced transport of oxygen and nutrients to and wastes away from the lower extremities. To remedy this problem, simply sleep with your legs and feet covered with an extra blanket.

Low blood sugar is another cause of leg cramps. Consequently, foods containing either concentrated sugar or large amounts of sugar should be avoided.

If you do get a cramp, try extending the involved muscles as soon as you feel the cramp begin. Walking on the cramped foot also helps. Take a mineral supplement containing calcium, magnesium, and a full spectrum of other minerals required for absorption. Mineral supplements in tablet form should be chewed thoroughly for prompt absorption and then washed down with some water.

MASSAGE THERAPY

Painful conditions of the muscles or joints usually involve muscular spasms. Overused or traumatized muscles produce lactic acid and other irritating waste products. These toxins cause nerves to transmit impulses that make the muscles contract. Even more waste products are then formed, preventing the flow of blood to remove these toxins and bring oxygen and nutrients. Thus, a vicious cycle is perpetuated. The muscles in spasm then can cause pain and abnormal, damaging pressure on joints.

One way to break this cycle is to ingest or rub in anti-inflammatory substances. Another way is massage. Natural movement often helps and can sometimes be facilitated by muscle relaxants and anti-inflammatory drugs.

There are a number of different massage systems such as Swedish massage, Shiatsu, Rolfing, etc. Swedish massage primarily involves rubbing of the skin with oil. Shiatsu involves precisely focused acupressure. Rolfing involves deep massage using strong pressure with the aim of dispersing memories of emotional traumas embedded in the musculature.

My one (unpleasant) experience with Rolfing was extremely painful, and I begged the woman doing the massage to apply less pressure. She assured me that the pain was emotional, not physical. However, afterward, I saw that the massaged parts of my body were visibly bruised. Shortly after the massage, I felt unable to deal appropriately with even slightly emotional situations, and this unpleasant after-effect lasted for about two days.

Since that experience and a few others, I am very selective in allowing anyone to do massage on me. However, there are many extraordinarily talented massage therapists, and you will know when you find the right one. Once you do, you should strive to have a complete massage at least monthly.

Leg and Ankle Massage

Those who practice T'ai-Chi movement or otherwise use their legs strenuously will inevitably experience muscle, tendon, or ligament strain. One of the most effective ways to relieve such strain is to thoroughly explore the painful region, find the focus of pain, and carefully massage that spot. It is important to use just the right pressure, for too much pressure can further traumatize the tissues involved. Also, during massage, the legs should be aligned so that the muscles in the region are in their most relaxed orientation. Massage brings blood, oxygen, ch'i, and nutrients to the region and assists in the removal of irritating waste products.

DIT DA JOW

Dit da jow is an herbal remedy for bruises and sprains. Its formulation is literally thousands of years old. Those interested in learning more about dit da jow are referred to two articles on the subject by Brian Gray.* Dit da jow is inexpensive and readily available in Chinese grocery or herb stores. If you live far from such stores, you can purchase a few versions of it from various mail-order martial arts supply companies.†

Dramatic relief occurs within a minute or two when dit da jow is promptly rubbed into a bruise or sprain. The value of dit da jow is not limited to mere pain relief; it also reduces swelling and inflammation, brings ch'i and blood to the area, and helps to remove waste products.

Some versions of dit da jow are considered safe to consume internally, but the stronger preparations are for external use only.

CH'I

Over the years, I have found that ch'i‡ can effectively remedy all manner of conditions including bruises, sprains, headaches, stopped-up nose, sore throat, and cuts. The sooner you apply ch'i to an injury, the shorter the recovery time. Ch'i is not a cure but assists the healing process; first aid or professional attention may still be required. For example, a cut should be kept clean and bandaged, and a broken bone must be set and immobilized.

The following two anecdotes illustrate applications of ch'i that are routine for me and other Ch'i Kung practitioners.

About twenty years ago, I injured a muscle in my thigh. It ached so much at night that I would awaken and need to get out of bed and move and massage it to relieve the pain. After a few months, I got the idea to send ch'i to the muscle without getting out of bed. The ch'i gave almost immediate and complete relief for the entire night. Finally, I reached the point where I would *literally* send the ch'i in my sleep.

As a physics teacher, I demonstrate to my students that I can place a seventeen-pound iron bar in my hand and hit it full force with a

---

*"Liquid Gold or Fool's Potion?" *Inside Kung Fu*, Vol. 19, No. 7, July, 1992 and "Dit Da Jow: Making Kung-Fu's Liquid Gold," *Inside Kung Fu,* Vol. 19, No. 10, October, 1992.

†BLT Supplies, Inc., 35-01 Queens Boulevard, Long Island City, NY 11101, 1-800-322-2860.

‡For more on ch'i, see Robert Chuckrow, *The Tai Chi Book*, YMAA Publication Center, Boston MA, 1998, Ch. 2, and Robert Chuckrow, *Introduction to Ch'i Kung* (videotape), Rising Mist Publications, PO Box 50, Briarcliff Manor, NY 10510.

one-pound hammer without injuring my hand. To make the demonstration more dramatic, I first pretend to enter a state of meditation and do some exaggerated Ch'i-Kung movements to "make my hand impervious to damage." Of course, afterward, I explain the underlying physical principle, which is that the hammer harmlessly bounces off the iron bar without transferring much energy. I also admit later that the Ch'i-Kung movements were unnecessary and just an act.

One year, after doing this demonstration and then explaining its harmlessness, a student wanted to try it. When I hit the bar with the hammer, he yelled in pain. At first, I thought it was a joke but saw that he was really hurt. His hand was starting to swell and change color. Evidently he had placed the bar on his knuckles instead of the soft part of his hand.

I immediately held my hand a few inches above the injury and began sending ch'i. My unconventional behavior prompted some giggles from some students in the class. I sternly told them that they needed to keep absolutely quiet. After about thirty seconds, the injured hand was normal, having full movement without pain.

At this point, he and the other students were keenly interested in knowing how I accomplished this change. After I explained ch'i as best I could, they wanted me to teach them to experience and send it. I replied that they needed to study T'ai Chi with me first. Within a week, the yearly T'ai-Chi class I teach as a physical education elective swelled to about two-dozen students. Also, students with minor injuries began coming to me for healing. Of course, I explained that, other than for close friends or members of my immediate family, I only send ch'i to injuries I have caused.

I have thought extensively about how ch'i makes pain subside so quickly. My reasoning is as follows: Pain is the way your body tells you that it is injured and needs constructive attention. When you are injured, the flow of ch'i is interrupted by fear and tension. Reinstating the flow greatly accelerates the healing process and, except for a serious injury, makes pain superfluous. So pain subsides.

Learning to send ch'i is easy and natural. Once you feel ch'i, you should practice sending it to any injury you may get, no matter how small. With practice, your skill (kung) will increase and may be indispensable if you are sick or seriously injured.

Sending healing ch'i should be done with caution, since it can be draining and even harmful. There should be no egotistical thoughts such as, "look at what I can do that others can't." The only thoughts should be (1) a pure motivation to help another person and (2) a visualization of energy entering your body from behind and being focused by you as if you were a lens. As just mentioned, I cautiously restrict my sending of ch'i only to those whom I have harmed (always inadvertently) or those with whom I have a loving or close relationship.

THERAPEUTIC MAGNETS

In Japan and other parts of the world, small, powerful magnets are available in drugstores. These magnets are used to relieve muscle spasms and chronic pain. The magnets are placed in contact with the painful region and held in place for a day or so with an adhesive bandage.

I know a number of people who swear that magnets have relieved and even cured their severe conditions of bursitis and even arthritis. Is there a scientific explanation for how the magnets work, if indeed they do? Consider the following interpretation based on simple physiology and elementary physics.

It is known that nerve impulses are electric currents and that electric currents are affected by magnetic fields. In particular, if a magnetic field is applied at right angles to a current, the current will be deflected in a direction perpendicular to both the directions of the current and the magnetic field.

Therapeutic magnets are commonly applied to the skin in such a way that their magnetic fields are directed perpendicularly to the surface. On the other hand, nerves usually travel parallel to the skin and, therefore, perpendicular to the applied magnetic field. Consequently, the currents comprising the nerve impulses would be deflected parallel to the skin but perpendicular to the length of the nerve. Thus, the affected nerve impulses should be inhibited. The result could well be that the vicious cycle of escalating nerve irritation and muscle tension is then broken, thus relieving the muscular spasm and its resulting pain and damage.

CHAPTER 12

The Importance of Aerobic Exercise in Weight Loss

IS T'AI CHI A TOTAL EXERCISE?

It is often said that T'ai Chi is a total exercise—that if you practice T'ai Chi daily, no other exercise is required for perfect health and optimal weight. Of course, this assertion is true but only if you consistently practice all aspects of T'ai Chi: empty-handed form, push-hands, sword, broadsword, staff, lance, two-person form, and sparring. How many T'ai-Chi players do any more than just the empty-handed form, which is extremely beneficial but non-aerobic? Not many. Most players who do push-hands practice it only once or twice a week, not daily. And then, how many push-hands players do highly spirited push-hands?

Exercise has many benefits and is a vast and varied subject about which many books have been written. Here, we will be mainly concerned with exercise as it pertains to weight loss. Chapter 14 contains a synopsis of some important aspects of running, the ultimate aerobic exercise aerobic exercise. The concepts discussed in Chapter 14 apply, of course, to many other exercises.

THE CONNECTION BETWEEN AEROBIC EXERCISE AND WEIGHT LOSS

An aerobic activity is one that raises the pulse rate for extended periods of time, so that oxygen utilization is trained to become more efficient.*† Some examples of aerobic exercises are running, swimming, cycling, rowing, and tennis. There is no question that aerobic exercise is important for weight loss. Whereas aerobic exercise is certainly important for weight loss, the reasons given for this benefit are usually

*See Kenneth H. Cooper, *Aerobics*, M. Evans and Company, Inc., New York, NY 1968, pp. 38–39.

†Also see Covert Bailey, *The New Fit or Fat*, Houghton Mifflen Co., Boston, MA 1991, pp. 54–59.

misleading or incorrect. Let us examine each claim in turn:

Claim 1. *Vigorous regular exercise can eventually increase muscle mass, and this long-term increase can raise the overall metabolism rate.*

This claim is probably true but only if exercise is done regularly and over a long period of time.

Claim 2. *During exercise, the body "burns more calories" than if the exercise were not done.*

To see the prevalence of this concept, just go to any fitness center and look at the information listed on the various machines. Many are equipped with a read-out of the number of calories burned, implying that a caloric expenditure during exercise meaningfully corresponds to a weight loss. In fact, the extra energy burned because of exercising is quite minor unless the exercise is extremely strenuous and done continuously for many hours. For example, only 73 calories,* (about that in a slice of bread) would be expended by a 180-pound person climbing to the top of the Empire State Building. Few are able to do sufficiently vigorous exercise long enough to burn a substantial amount of energy.

Claim 3. *For a sustained period after exercise, the body burns additional calories.*

Exercising regularly makes it easier to lose weight, which makes it seem reasonable that exercise causes a prolonged increase in metabolism rate. There is, however, no proof of any increase in metabolism rate for any substantial period after a session of exercise.

The following is what appears to be the true relationship of exercise to weight loss:

The function of aerobic exercise in a weight-loss program is not so much to burn energy as to change the way the body utilizes its energy reserves.†

That is, aerobic exercise teaches the body to burn fat rather than sugar. Here is how:

Sustained exertion requires the muscles to expend energy, which comes from three sources. One source is stored glycogen that is changed back to sugar by means of epinephrine. Another source is stored fat. The third source is the conversion of muscle protein into glucose, which can be burned (gluconeogenesis).‡

---

*Considering that a pound of fat contains 3,500 calories, 73 calories corresponds to a loss of fat equaling only 1/3 ounce!

†The only book I have been able to find that emphatically corroborates this concept is Covert Bailey, *Fit or Fat*, Houghton Mifflin Co. Boston, MA, 1978.

‡See W.D. McArdle, F.I. Katch, and V. L. Katch, *Exercise Physiology*, Lea & Febiger, Philadelphia, PA 1986, pp. 8–11.

The stores of glycogen are limited and can be depleted with extended exertion. Glycogen depletion causes a drop in blood sugar. Because the brain and vital organs require a certain level of blood sugar, the body takes steps to ensure that the level of blood sugar does not get too low. Where can this sugar come from? One might think that it can come from fat. Certainly, excess sugar is turned into stores of fat. However, while sugar can be changed to fat, fat can not easily be changed back to sugar. Whereas protein *can* be and is easily converted to sugar, substantial conversion is undesirable because it is at the expense of vital muscle tissue. Thus, frequent, sustained exertion places pressure on the body to burn fat more readily.

Consider running. Unless you run non-stop for very long periods, it is unlikely that *all* of the glycogen stores of your body will be depleted. However, locally accessible stores of glycogen within the calf and thigh muscles *may* be substantially depleted during a thirty-minute period of running. Therefore, such extended vigorous muscular activity places a pressure on the body to use glycogen as sparingly as possible. Repetition of such activity trains the body to improve its efficiency in utilizing stores of fat and to use as little glycogen as possible. Also, the body learns to store increased quantities of accessible glycogen to prevent a "glycogen famine." Except when a seasoned runner is under unusual stress, glycogen levels tend not to be depleted, and the body comfortably utilizes fat for energy. Thus, low blood sugar and its consequent hunger are infrequent. In short, running and other aerobic exercises teach the body to comfortably burn excess fat and go for relatively long periods without hunger.

By combining prolonged exercise with sensible nutrition and supplementation, you can change your metabolism from utilization of sugar to utilization of fat. Then you will become a person who tends not to become fat.

If a fat burner eats a large quantity of carbohydrate in a short period of time, more of this carbohydrate can be stored as glycogen rather than as fat because the glycogen storage capacity is large. Whatever *is* stored as fat is later burned in a routine fashion. The body tries to conserve or increase fat reserves only when the stores of fat become so low that they threaten to be insufficient.

Notice that it is not that a person who runs burns more energy and thus loses weight. Rather, the runner is better at burning fat than someone who does not run. An inconsequential amount of additional energy is burned during exercise and for a short period afterward. However, the effect on the manner in which energy is utilized is crucial.

By contrast, the following happens to people who lead a sedentary life: glycogen storage is small, and the muscles prefer to use glycogen for energy rather than fat. After short amounts of daily activity, glycogen reserves drop and low blood sugar occurs, with a consequent craving for refined carbohydrate. Carbohydrate is then usually eaten in excess of the limited glycogen-storage capacity of the body. The carbohydrate that cannot be stored as glycogen is then converted to fat and stored. However, this fat is never burned. It remains. Thus, a sedentary person will constantly crave food, continue to gain weight easily, and have a difficult time losing weight. If weight *is* lost, that weight—and more—will most likely be regained.

CHAPTER 13

Miscellaneous

THE POWER OF THE MIND

The mind has the ability to isolate and focus on a detail so intently that, for all practical purposes, nothing else in the world exists. Or, it can blank out thoughts, information, and sensory data. The ability to focus or not is neutral—neither good nor bad. How it is applied is a different matter. If the mind isolates and focuses on a negative thought, memory, or feeling, the result can be failure, pain, and even damage to oneself or others. Similar consequences can occur if important events are disregarded. Conversely, achievements of the highest kind are possible when the mind focuses on a constructive enterprise or eliminates the perception of interfering factors. That is why every thought and everything that is said must be self-monitored. All negativity must be cleaned out.

USE OF PERSONAL SOUND DEVICES WHILE WALKING

We are living in an era of expectation of immediate gratification and almost constant overstimulation. Whatever is considered desirable must be instantly available—often to an excessive degree. We have electric light at night, fast food when we are hungry, the ability to instantly communicate with others half way around the world, next-day delivery of any purchase, entertainment of all sorts at all hours of the day or night on television, projections of election results long before the votes are counted, and privately heard music wherever we go.

Our societal need for around-the-clock stimulation and frequent overstimulation stems from a sense of emptiness. Many of us have lost our connection with nature, have no way of fulfilling our creative potential, and do not know the joy of uplifting others and ourselves. The void created by not having access to these basic expressions of our spiritual destiny cannot be filled by external stimulation. Therefore, the substitutes, which are usually meaningless sources of excitement, need to be ever-present and constantly escalated in intensity.

The addition of music is superfluous when the mind is thoroughly in the moment and involved in creative and spiritual endeavors or communing with nature.

Another negative aspect of listening to music while walking outdoors is that it increases vulnerability to automobiles and human and animal predators. While outside, it is essential to observe and be totally aware of everything that can result in personal harm.

There is a time and place to listen to music. When we listen to music while walking outdoors, eating, making love, etc., our attention to either activity is divided. Listening to uplifting, inspired music and communing with nature should be separate experiences, each requiring total attentiveness. Uninspired music is not worth listening to.

CARRYING THINGS

At times, you may need to carry items carrying things ranging from minute to bulky. You may find that even small items in your pants pockets are quite uncomfortable. Depending on how much you need to carry, you will find that most clothing and camping equipment stores carry a variety of backpacks, shoulder bags, and hip packs. You may find that carrying a weight on your hip is less of a strain on your back than carrying it higher up.

A folding all-purpose luggage cart (see Fig. 13-1), available in department stores for about $20, is indispensable for hauling heavy items over long distances. If you purchase such a cart, select the one with the largest wheels. It is also a good idea to remove the wheels

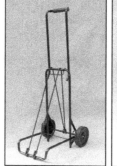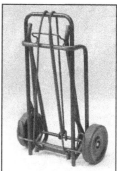

Fig. 13-1. *Folding luggage cart, opened and folded.*

and apply a coating of grease or petroleum jelly to the axles. Lubrication is usually absent.

OPENING DOORS

Have you ever tried to push a door open just as someone simultaneously pulls it open from the other side? If you are over-committed to the action, you fall forward. You should strive to reach the point where your balance is not even slightly disrupted when doors unexpectedly recede.

ORIENTING YOURSELF WHEN LOST AT NIGHT

A few months ago I became lost late at night while driving my car. The area was near a very irregular coastline of Long Island Sound, and I became very confused. Each time I drove away from the water, I saw water in the opposite direction. I had no street map and no compass.

I got out of my car and looked at the sky. There were practically no stars out, and the north star was nowhere to be seen. By looking at the moon and taking into account its phase and the approximate time of day, I was able to orient myself. In a short time, I was back in a familiar area.

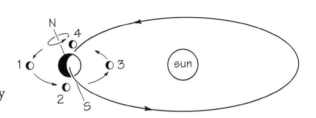

Fig. 13-2. *Relative positions of the sun, earth, and moon, shown in four representative positions. For the orientation of the earth shown, the northern hemisphere tilts away from the sun and, thus, is in winter.*

The trick is visualizing the relationship of the earth, sun, and moon or memorizing a few basic facts. The moon rotates about the earth in approximately the same plane as that of the earth* about the sun (see Fig 13-2). The earth rotates about its axis once per day, and this daily rotation, the monthly rotation of the moon about the earth, and the yearly rotation of the earth about the sun are all in the same direction. Because of the daily rotation of the earth about its axis, both the sun and moon rise in the east and set in the west. In the north temperate zone, both the sun and the moon are always in the south—more so during winter than summer.

The monthly rotation of the moon around the earth is in the same direction as that of the daily rotation of the earth on its axis. Therefore, when viewed at the same time of night, the position of the moon in the sky is displaced eastward from each day to the next.

When the moon is full (position 1 in Fig. 13-2), it is in the opposite direction of the sun and rises shortly after the sun sets. Every day

*Actually, the plane of the motion of the moon about the earth is tilted about 5 degrees with respect to the plane of the motion of the earth about the sun.

thereafter, the moon rises and sets roughly an hour later, until after about one week, it rises about midnight (last quarter, position 2) . Two weeks after it is full, it rises and sets about the same time as the sun. Now the moon is new (position 3). Every day thereafter, the moon rises and sets roughly an hour later, until after about two weeks, it is again full.

Shortly after the moon is new, it can be seen following the sun across the sky. Because the light from the sun illuminates the bright part of the crescent, the horns of the crescent moon face away from the sun. Shortly after the sun sets, the crescent moon is seen, horns-up, in the western sky. The crescent moon in this orientation resembles a bowl, which increasingly fills, night after night.

When the moon becomes half full (first quarter), it is highest in the sky around sunset, with the illuminated half facing the setting sun. The half moon sets about midnight.

As the moon approaches full, it lags more and more behind the sun until, when full, it rises just after the sun sets. Correspondingly, the full moon sets just before sunrise. Thereafter, the moon rises later and later. Now the waning moon appears to be followed by the sun, getting closer and closer every day. The moon now sets during the early morning, and the lit part faces the east.

When the moon becomes half full in the last quarter, it rises around midnight, is highest in the sky when the sun is rising, and sets around noon.

As the moon approaches new, it rises later and later in the morning, and the sun seems to be catching up with it. The illuminated half, of course, faces the sun, and the horns point away from the sun, toward the west. In this phase, the moon sets just before the sun and does not rise until slightly before dawn. The setting moon has its horns pointed downward, suggesting that it is an inverted bowl and, thus, emptying.

If you keep track of the phases of the moon, you should be able to know the time and the direction of north whenever the moon is out.

CHAPTER 14

T'ai-Chi Running

Whereas swimming, cycling, rowing, and tennis are excellent aerobic exercises, running is the only one requiring no equipment or special facilities—just oneself. Running is considered by many experts on cardiovascular fitness to yield the maximum benefit in the shortest time. However, the benefits, cautions, and concepts mentioned in this chapter apply not only to running but can be extended to *any* aerobic exercise.

I can remember the era when the few people who ran were considered eccentric by the general public. In time, running became a fad whose virtues were extolled. At present, running is again spurned. Health-care professionals warn runners that the endorphin rush they experience from running can actually become addictive, leading them to push themselves far beyond healthy exertion. Running is said to be bad for the knees, ankles, tendons, spine, and internal organs. People are encouraged to walk, not run. Many do fast walking or use expensive exercise machines.

Of course, injury can occur when any beneficial activity is done incorrectly. The answer is not to avoid running but to learn to run correctly.

Running is natural. Our bodies are beautifully designed for locomotion over a wide range of speeds. Physiologically, we are not that different from other animals that run for hours a day just for the sheer joy of it. As with many valuable things, running can be harmful when misunderstood and incorrectly done. Oversimplifying running—or any activity, for that matter—deprives us of its potential benefits.

We get into trouble while running, not because running is bad but because we misunderstand how our bodies work anatomically. Many of us have developed harmful movement patterns, which take their toll after many repetitions. Then we disregard and misinterpret the warning signs when we exceed our limitations.

Running can provide substantial health benefits and improved physical and mental self-understanding for people when they learn to use their bodies correctly.

BENEFITS OF CORRECT RUNNING

Cardiovascular. One well-known benefit is improved tone, strength, and endurance of the entire cardiovascular system. Another benefit is that almost all the bones and muscles of the body are strengthened by running.

Elimination of Toxins. During running, the body temperature rises as high as four Fahrenheit degrees above normal. This rise indicates stepped-up activity of the eliminative organs and a corresponding stepped-up flushing out of poisons through perspiration. However, the high temperature does *not* produce the discomfort normally accompanying a fever of the same temperature. On the contrary, there is a sense of well-being, and the accompanying stimulation of the brain is very beneficial and enjoyable.

Increased Adaptation to and Recovery from Stress. With time, the efficiency of the circulatory system increases, and the oxygenating, nourishing, and cleansing effects of the blood are more readily available to all the tissues of the body. Thus, the body is able to produce a larger and more-sustained energy output when needed.

Changes in Fat Metabolism. Those who run regularly often experience a beneficial loss of weight and are not perpetually hungry. The mechanism for this benefit is usually attributed to an adaptation of the body to the demands of running by becoming more trim and, consequently, more efficient. It is also asserted that the caloric requirements of aerobic exercise are responsible for the weight loss. In Chapter 12, the weight loss from aerobic exercise is explained by offering a mechanism by which it helps transform a person who is a sugar burner into a fat burner.

Improved Efficiency and Coordination of Movement. With each step during running, the musculature of the whole body is called upon to maintain stability while the muscles of the legs strenuously move throughout their range. When running is done with awareness, the nervous system is activated and trained with every step.

Other Benefits. Running massages organs and glands, cleanses the lungs, improves vital capacity (the maximum amount of air that can be exhaled in one breath), assists the circulation of lymph, and results in a sense of elation and well-being.

DANGERS OF INCORRECT RUNNING

Over the past two decades, I have observed that an alarming number of runners harm their knees, feet, ankles, breasts, and internal organs. Many runners cave in their arches and, consequently, place harmful shearing stress on their knees with each step.

Incorrect Alignment. When alignment is correct, muscles designed for the task of stabilizing the body during movement are naturally brought into play. Also, joints are subjected to compressive forces, which they are designed to withstand. However, when alignment is faulty, weaker muscles, not designed to do the job of stronger ones, are subjected to severe stress, which can cause damage to those muscles and their tendons (tendons connect muscles to bones). When repeated stress is exerted on joints in an extreme placement, danger to ligaments and joints increases. There are two harmful effects: (1) pressures are placed on cartilage in locations where it is thin, thereby wearing it down. (2) When joints are not centered, they are subject to large amounts of leverage. Chronically stressed ligaments can stretch or tear when subjected to a sudden movement (ligaments are bands of fibrous tissue that keep joints from dislocating). Being overweight intensifies the ill effects of poor alignment. The solution is not to cut out running altogether but only until you correct your alignment and lose weight.

There seems to be a widespread reluctance to accept that alignment can be changed. During the years that I have been teaching movement, I have many times heard students say with respect to their incorrect alignment, "That's the way I am," or, "That's the way I was born." In the words of one of my teachers, Elaine Summers, I reply, "No, that's the way you are *wearing* your body." Unfortunately, many find it quite difficult to change alignment—not because of an inability of the tissues involved to change but from a mental attachment to a particular pattern of use. There must be a strong motivation to change, combined with perseverance and a knowledgeable teacher.

Consider an excessive forward curvature of the spine in the waist area ("swayback"). Here the muscles on the inside of the spine are extended to an extreme of their range, and the opposing muscles (on the outside of the spine) are excessively contracted. Rather than being centered with respect to each other, the vertebrae are situated with excess pressure toward the rear of each. This pressure causes a distortion of the discs, which can become permanent. This incorrect alignment is certainly bad enough during standing, sitting, and walking but can create a serious problem when combined with the repeated stress produced by the impact of each step of running.

The lower the part of the body, the more critical the effect of incorrect alignment. For example, the knees bear almost the entire body weight, while the feet bear the entire weight. The knees and the arches of the feet are both shock absorbers. When the alignment of these is off, not only does direct harm result to the knees and feet, but also their shock-absorbing function is impaired, increasing shock to all parts of the body.

When the arch caves in, the ankle joint moves away from center, causing it to be easily injured. Likewise, when a knee buckles inward, it, too, is very vulnerable to injury. Many knee problems result from habitually caving in the arches and knees. Poor ankle/knee alignment is quite common and usually starts at an early age. However long a person has had undesirable habits, with proper understanding and diligent practice, it is possible to eliminate them in only a few weeks.*

Methods of attaining the correct alignment of the feet and knees have been discussed in Chapter 3. Here, again, is how to experience the proper lateral alignment of the arches, ankles and knees: Stand with feet parallel and directly below the thigh joints (centerlines of feet about 9 in. apart). Alternately move the weight from the outsides of the feet to the insides, taking smaller and smaller excursions away from center. Alignment will be correct when the center of the weight distribution on each foot is centered on each foot.

Harmful Impact to the Body. The runner must be careful not to produce jarring impact but, instead, absorb it. Remember, the harmful effects of any incorrect alignment are exacerbated by forceful impact and reduced by lessening the jarring effects of vertical motion of the body. This reduction involves a natural flexing of the arches, ankles, knees, and spine, which are shock absorbers.

Another injurious result of excessive impact is the repeated stress on tissues, which become stretched by the combined effect of their weight and jarring up-and-down motion. Breasts, internal organs, and skin (including facial skin) can be stretched and caused to sag by repeated

*For a detailed treatment of alignment of knees, ankles, and arches, see Robert Chuckrow, *The Tai Chi Book*, YMAA Publication Center, Boston, MA, 1998, Ch. 5.

impact. People who suffer from hernias and prolapsed uteruses must be especially cautious.

Strain on the Heart. The heart is a muscle that needs to be supplied with oxygenated blood—especially when demands are made on it. At a certain level of stress, the blood supply to the heart may be insufficient for its level of activity. This occurrence is called a *myocardial insufficiency.* If the insufficiency continues for an extended period of time, tissue damage can occur, resulting in a *myocardial infarction* (heart attack).

Exertion should be gradually and cautiously raised from very mild to appropriately strenuous. Rather than suddenly increasing the exertion on a particular day when a burst of energy is felt, save part of this excess energy for the next day. Gentle but consistent running is better than sporadic bursts of high output. See "Other Important Considerations For Aerobic Exercise," later in this chapter, for commonly accepted criteria for target heart rates.

Inadequate Nutrition. Since any vigorous exercise taxes the heart, it is wise to take supplements of minerals required for proper heart function, namely, selenium, calcium, magnesium, zinc, etc. Additionally, vitamins E and C improve the efficiency of the circulatory system. Most food is grown on devitalized soil, and then most of its vitamins and minerals are removed during the refining process. Thus, whether or not we do vigorous exercise, we need to take vitamin and mineral supplements.* Alcohol and sweets other than fresh fruit should be totally avoided. These substances deplete the body of valuable nutrients and lower the motivation for exercise.

Dehydration. One frequently mentioned danger is that of dehydration on a very hot, humid day. It is a good idea to drink an ample quantity of water about fifteen minutes before running in anticipation of a corresponding loss later.

Electrolyte Imbalance. Electrolyte imbalance is definitely possible and a serious condition. Later in this chapter, we will discuss aspects of dietary salt and explain why an electrolyte imbalance is more likely to occur in those with a high intake of salt.

Overzealousness. Runners who start to experience the benefits of running sometimes overdo it. One of my T'ai-Chi students ran competitively when he was in college. At that time he ran as much as fifteen

*For suggested daily supplementation, see Gary Price Todd, M.D., *Nutrition, Health, & Disease,* Whitford Press, West Chester, PA,1985, pp.193–194.

miles per day. He said, "Something wonderful happens when you run fifteen miles that doesn't happen when you run two or three miles." However, his sustained running in very cold weather had damaged his knee joints. Now he has stopped running altogether. Would it not have been better for him to run shorter distances or skip running altogether on days when the weather was so extreme instead of pushing himself beyond normal limitations and injuring himself?

Competitiveness. Another problem is that of competitiveness. Competitiveness—even if it is with yourself—clouds judgment when it comes to safety. The impulse to win or to better your time jeopardizes the most valid reason for doing anything, namely, to improve health and understanding. For example, don't be embarrassed about alternating walking and running if you become winded. Above all, walk if pain occurs. It may signal a serious problem.

Last, timing yourself should only be used to measure progress over a period of time much longer than a few days. You should progress at the rate that feels best instead of setting unrealistic goals for yourself. Satisfying such goals may require damaging exertion and lead to a setback. Stay in touch with your body.

OTHER IMPORTANT CONSIDERATIONS FOR AEROBIC EXERCISE

Warm-up and Stretching. A proper warm-up before any strenuous activity—especially running—is indispensable. A good motto is, "if you don't have time to stretch, then you don't have time to run." Warming up should not tax or strain any part of your body. Moving cautiously and gently helps to distribute the synovial fluid (the oil that lubricates the joints) over the surfaces of the joints. Moreover, the ligaments, which keep the moving surfaces in proper alignment, are given gentle stress in preparation for more strenuous demands later.

First move the wrists, ankles, head, hip joints, shoulder joints, vertebrae, and knees throughout their range without any strain whatsoever. Next extend muscles without any resistance of opposing muscles, gravity, or momentum produced by "bouncing." Then, the predictable and constant pull of gravity, combined with a judiciously chosen degree of leverage can be utilized to slowly stretch the muscles further. Only when the muscles are sufficiently prepared is it permissible to bounce, utilizing momentum and gravity for a final tone-up.

After stretching, the cardiovascular system should be activated only through movement of escalating speed. It is essential to allow sufficient time for the heart and blood vessels to adapt and for the blood to naturally thin in preparation for a higher flow rate.

The runner should gradually increase speed over a period of about twenty minutes or more, depending upon the messages sent by the body. It is best to begin with walking, then faster walking, and finally slow running alternated with walking until the body craves running without rest. It takes a while for the blood to become thin enough for heavy exertion to be safe.*

Heart Rate. It is good to take your pulse on a regular basis. As you become more attuned to your body, you will know when your heart is beating too fast. You can rest your heart by walking slowly. If you overuse a muscle it can be a problem, but if that muscle is your heart then the problem will be much greater.

The following are commonly accepted criteria for maximum and target heart rates during aerobic exercise:†

Maximum allowable heart rate = 220 − age.

For example, for a person aged 35, the maximum allowable heart rate is 220 − 35 = 185. The actual (target) heart rate during exercise should be kept well below this rate. A conservative criterion is to sustain the heart rate within 65% to 80% of the maximum. For a person aged 35, the suggested target range is calculated to be 120 to 148 beats per minute. Those in top condition can achieve a target rate of 85%, but in no event should they exceed 90%.

No matter what the suggested criteria are, you should always avoid becoming distressfully out of breath. Additionally, it is a bad sign when a high pulse rate does not drop after more than a minute or two of rest. At the beginning, you may experience cardiac, respiratory, or muscular discomfort before you reach the target range. As the condition of your muscles and respiratory and circulatory systems improve, it will become easier for you to sustain the target rate comfortably.

Those with a history of heart or circulatory problems or who suspect that they may have such problems should consult a cardiologist before

---

*For more on warm-up and stretching, see Chapter 6 of the *The Tai Chi Book*.

†See W.D. McArdle, F.I. Katch, and V. L. Katch, *Exercise Physiology*, Lea & Febiger, Philadelphia, PA 1986, pp.358–359.

undertaking any aerobic or otherwise vigorous activity. It might be wise to do so even if no problem seems evident.

Pausing to Rest and Allow Ch'i to Circulate. About fifteen years ago, I joined a local aerobics class. Midway through the first class, I felt that I was over-exerting myself and stopped to rest. The leader of the class then said, "Robert, the worst thing you can do is suddenly stop the movement in the middle of the class. It could give you a heart attack." I went back to the movement even though the class was extremely fast-paced and strenuous. The next day, my leg muscles were very sore, and the pain lasted for days. A week later, just before the start of the next class, a woman asked the leader, "After last week's class, my legs were so sore that I couldn't walk for almost a week. Is that normal?" The leader replied that it *was* normal, saying, "You'll get past that after a while." Right then I decided that, if I got tired during class, I would just stop and rest.

Again, midway through the class, I started to feel that it was too much. I walked over to a large table and lay down on my back. The leader then said, "Robert, if you stop now, you can have a heart attack." I resolutely asserted that I would take responsibility for any consequent harm. As I lay there, I was amazed at the degree to which ch'i was circulating throughout my body. I knew that it was not the room because I had taught T'ai Chi in that very room for years and was very familiar with its energy. After about five minutes, I eased back into the class and was again amazed at my increased vitality as a result of that short rest.

The combination of T'ai Chi practice and running is one of the best I have ever found. Whenever I go running, I periodically pause and reap the benefit of resting and feeling the resulting heightened flow of ch'i. Sometimes I stop under a tree and do Ch'i Kung. Other times I do a round of the T'ai-Chi form. Even though I certainly do not do competitive running and never push myself to the limit, I am, nevertheless, careful to gradually and continuously change from relatively high exertion down to a calm, meditative state before starting Ch'i Kung practice.

In recent years, I have been doing very spirited, aerobic push-hands practice. Here too, alternating push-hands with Ch'i Kung or the T'ai-Chi form gives me not only that wonderful boost in energy but also helps me to regain a state of *sung* so necessary for proper push-hands practice.

Clean Air. Much of the benefit from running is negated by deeply breathing automotive exhaust fumes. Breathing clean air is crucial. Always avoid running near traffic or whenever the air is noticeably polluted.

Breathing. To flush stale air from the lungs, it is necessary to exhale fully. Runners should practice increasing the depth of their exhalations.* In order to fill the lungs with fresh air, the lungs need to empty first. Additionally, inhalations should be through the nose as much as is possible. The nasal passages should be cleansed to permit their optimal humidification and filtering of the air.†

The Need for Salt. There is no question that the two elements, sodium and chlorine, of which salt is composed, are necessary in human nutrition. However, these elements should be present in sufficient quantities in natural foods such as fruits, vegetables, grains, nuts, and seeds. Why then do people desire to consume many times as much salt as would be naturally present, and why is there the widespread belief that salt pills are needed in the summer? The answer can be very simply stated (although it requires elaboration); namely, *salt is genuinely addictive.* An addiction to a drug is defined as a "habituation to the use of a drug, the deprivation of which gives rise to symptoms of distress, abstinence, or withdrawal symptoms, and an irresistible impulsion to take the drug again."‡ This definition can be extended to nutrients by replacing the word *drug* in the above definition with the phrase *a nutrient in amounts substantially exceeding an optimal physiological requirement.*

The Harmful Effects of Salt. Because excess salt in the diet has been associated with high blood pressure, people feel that if their blood pressure is normal, no limitation of salt is required. There are, however, a number of reasons that *everyone* should limit salt intake.

1. **Flexibility of Muscles.** Every 9 grams of sodium chloride in body tissues binds one liter of water, which weighs over 2 pounds! Aside from its extra weight, that water clogs the tissues, thereby reducing flexibility of muscles. If you have ever experienced even minor swelling of your hands, you know

---

*The ability to move out stale air is termed *vital capacity,* which can be defined as the maximum amount of a full breath of air that can be expelled in a complete inhalation.

†For more on breathing, see Robert Chuckrow, *The Tai Chi Book*, YMAA Publication Center, Boston, MA, 1998, Ch. 4.

‡Stedman's Medical Dictionary, The Williams & Wilkinson Co., Baltimore, MD, 1966.

how stiff your fingers become. Just think of how any extra water must limit the flexibility of all of your muscles— including those used to focus the eyes on near and far objects.

2. **Strain on the Eliminative System.** All the excess salt you eat must be eliminated from the body. During cool weather, the burden falls mainly on the kidneys. During hot weather, the sweat glands are also actively involved in removing salt. Why make things more difficult for eliminative organs and glands that are already strained by other factors such as pollutants and pesticides?

3. **Impaired Digestion of Food.** The presence of salt in food inhibits sufficient chewing. Just notice the degree to which you tend to prematurely swallow food that has been salted. Salt added to food leads to drinking with and after meals. Consuming water while food is in the process of being digested dilutes the digestive juices and impairs digestion.

4. **Obstacles to Weight Loss.** Because salt taken in excess becomes addictive, there is a craving for salt when it is expelled from the body. When weight is lost, it is usually accompanied by a release of salt. In addition, the reduction of caloric intake required for weight loss usually means a lower salt intake. The result is a craving for salt. Because salt is associated with the foods containing it, there is usually a craving for these foods. The self-discipline required to resist these cravings is easier to muster when the above mechanism is kept in mind. That is, such cravings are a sign of progress and disappear as the body stabilizes.

   Retention of salt and its corresponding water can produce a weight gain without any change in the amount of body fat. Of course, the weight loss associated with the release of salt and its retained water is desirable but should not be misconstrued as resulting from a loss of fat.

5. **Susceptibility to Electrolyte Imbalance.** When the kidneys remove salt from the body, they "know" when to stop. That is, the kidneys normally will not remove so much salt from the blood that an electrolyte imbalance occurs. The sweat glands, however, do not know when to stop and can cause an imbalance.

If you consistently eat a lot of salt and then do heavy exercise in a hot, high-humidity environment, you may suffer a serious imbalance requiring some sort of replenishment. Whereas the ultimate answer is to gradually phase out excessive dietary salt, you must remedy an acute electrolyte imbalance promptly. The main symptoms of such an imbalance are abdominal cramps and nausea. If you do feel the need to replenish sodium after heavy exercise in hot weather, resist the urge to buy commercial sports drinks, which contain artificial color and other objectionable ingredients. Just stir a small amount of salt in some orange juice diluted with water. This natural version of a sports drink should do everything the commercial drinks will do without the phony stuff.

In the absence of symptoms of electrolyte imbalance, it is best to gradually clear the body of excess salt by tapering it out of the diet over a period of months or longer. Eventually your perspiration will be almost like water—essentially free of salt. When your perspiration has no salty taste, it is a sign that your body no longer is excreting an excess of salt. As long as the perspiration is salty, so much salt may be eliminated during profuse sweating that a sodium-potassium imbalance can occur. As the excess is eliminated, such danger becomes decreasingly likely.

Why Is Lowering Salt Intake Difficult? When too little salt is added to food, it is easy to remedy this deficiency by merely sprinkling some on. When too much salt has been added in preparation, it is impossible to remove without specialized equipment. We do not like to waste food, and if it is over-salted to our taste, we tend to eat it anyway. Therefore, people consume more salt than they would select to consume. Thus we become habituated to the taste of salt in our food. When food without salt is eaten, it has an unfamiliar taste. Habit makes it difficult for us to experiment with using less salt than we are used to.

How to Reduce Dietary Salt. It is very important to reduce dietary salt *gradually*. Prepare foods without adding any salt or using any ingredients containing added salt. Eat a few bites, chewing as long as possible. You may find that the taste is alien, but that is how any change initially feels. Soon, you will begin to taste the true flavor of the food. Then, after you have given the food a bit of a chance, add salt. Over time, reduce the amount of salt to a minute sprinkle. You will be surprised at how little salt it will now take to satisfy you.

Interpret any craving for salt as the body's withdrawal symptoms caused by its attempts to eliminate an excess. As the body gradually adapts, your interest in salt will continually diminish. Eventually, anything beyond a relatively small amount of salt will be distasteful.

Caution About Insufficient Dietary Salt. Do not try to completely eliminate added dietary salt. Remember that these days, many vegetables are deficient in natural minerals including sodium. You may occasionally need to sprinkle a small amount of salt on your food.

Exercising on an Empty Stomach. Strenuous exercise should always be done on an empty stomach. During digestion, the blood is directed to the digestive organs. Digestion involves (a) glandular secretions produced from nutrients supplied by the blood and (b) muscular contractions requiring stepped-up circulation of blood to the stomach. Thus, after a meal, the amount of blood available to the brain, heart, internal organs, and skeletal muscles is reduced. An insufficiency to the heart can be very dangerous.

Eating After Exercise. If a heavy meal is taken after running, the body is required to engage in the digestion of food rather than moving waste products from the muscles to the organs of elimination. If you are hungry after running, first restore body fluids by drinking pure water. Otherwise, you will be thirsty after consuming food. After the water is absorbed, eat fresh fruit such as an orange, chewing it thoroughly and slowly.

Experiment by paying close attention to the effects over a twenty-four-hour period of either eating or not eating soon after intense exercise. Note the quality of your sleep, the presence or absence of subsequent soreness, and the degree to which you sense a feeling of well-being.

Proper Footwear. Footwear for running should fit well, breathe, and cushion the heels and soles. There are numerous excellent brands on the market.

Running Surface. A varied natural surface is the most interesting. Running on concrete should be avoided whenever possible.

Cool-Down. Just as it is important to give the body time to adapt to vigorous activity, it is also important not to stop abruptly. After running, it is wise to spend the last ten minutes or more walking. During running, the blood vessels in the legs assist the action of the heart in pumping blood. If vigorous running is abruptly stopped, the heart may suddenly be overburdened. Also, do not sit for any length of time during the next few hours. Muscular movement helps the circulatory system to remove accumulated waste products.

Running on a Track. If you must use a track, try alternating clockwise and counterclockwise directions. Running with the curve of the track always to one side causes an unbalanced use of the body. Also, try running backward for a while to balance the use of muscles.

Frequency and Duration. Vigorous exercise should be interspersed with one or two days of rest per week. Some of the symptoms of overdoing running are muscle soreness, fatigue later in the day, and a restless night's sleep. The optimal frequency and distance will vary. Therefore, it is best not to hold any preconceived idea in this regard.

Walking. There has been a recent swing from running toward "low-impact" exercises. Walking is definitely more appropriate than running for elderly, obese, or very out of shape people or for those who have injuries or as-yet uncorrected alignment problems. However, for those in relatively good physical condition, walking must be very brisk or done in hilly terrain in order to yield any substantial benefit. For them, running is feasible if done with proper alignment, minimal impact, and common sense.

Until recently, the medical profession has disparaged the importance of exercise and diet. This attitude has been changing as people have begun to take more responsibility for their own health. However, few physicians have the time or training to instruct patients how to run without danger of injury. Their concept of health is based on traditional interpretation of statistical data. For example, if a cardiac patient can improve to the point that a heart attack becomes statistically unlikely, then nutrition and exercise conferring further benefits is often neglected. Only during the last few years have a handful of physicians begun to research and publish findings about diet and exercise that can guide patients to higher levels of physical development. There are levels of health beyond not having heart attacks, just as there are levels of nutritional well-being beyond not manifesting symptoms of nutrition-deficiency diseases.

Therefore, the differences between running and walking should not be considered just in terms of avoiding a heart attack. There are a number of important benefits of running that cannot be obtained by walking. Some of these benefits are the ability to adjust to a sustained high level of activity, elevation of body temperature, deep breathing, training the system to absorb and utilize large quantities of oxygen, and training the body to burn fat instead of sugar.

An Interesting Visual Illusion. See if you, too, experience the following illusion: When you stop after running for a long time, look at the sky. Notice that the clouds seem to be constantly receding. During running, the visual size of objects you are approaching is constantly increasing. Evidently the mind corrects for this increase and temporarily continues when you stop running. You then perceive the size of clouds to be decreasing. The sky then appears to be receding.

In Closing. Watch people. Observe their idiosyncrasies, faults, and strengths. See what you can learn from them. Then, look at yourself, and work on improving. You will find that as you continue in your quest for self-development, you will become more productive, open-minded, self-reliant, and creative. You will then naturally assist others to be likewise.

Bibliography

Ahn, Don, *Power Food: Food for Energy and Healing from the Taoist Tradition*, Ahn Tai Chi Studios, P.O. Box 301 Canal Street Station, New York, NY 10013, Videotape. 1986.

Aihara Herman, *Acid and Alkaline*, George Ohsawa Macrobiotic Foundation, Oroville, CA, 1976.

Ashley, Clifford W., *The Ashley Book of Knots*, Doubleday & Company, Garden City, NY, 1944.

Bailey, Covert, *Fit or Fat?*, Houghton Mifflin Co. Boston, MA, 1978.

Bailey, Covert, *The New Fit or Fat*, Houghton Mifflin Co. Boston, MA, 1991.

Bukkyo Dendo Kyokai (Buddhist Promoting Foundation), *The Teaching of Buddha*, 3-14, 4-chome, Shiba, Minato-ku, Tokyo, Japan, T108, 1980.

Chang, Dr. Stephen T., *The Complete System of Self-Healing Internal Exercises*, Tao Publishing Co., San Francisco, CA, 1986.

Chuckrow, Robert, *Introduction to Ch'i Kung*, Rising Mist Publications, PO Box 50, Briarcliff Manor, NY 10510. Videotape.

Chuckrow, Robert, *The Intelligent Dieter's Guide*, Rising Mist Publications, PO Box 50, Briarcliff Manor, NY 10510, 1997.

Chuckrow, Robert, *The Tai Chi Book*, YMAA Publication Center, Boston, MA, 1998.

Cooper, Kenneth, *Aerobics*, M. Evans and Company, Inc., New York, 1968.

Corbett, Margaret Darst, *Help Yourself to Better Sight*, Prentice-Hall, Inc., Englewood Cliffs, NJ, 1949.

Daniels, Farrington Jr., van der Leun, Jan C., and Johnson, Brian E., "Sunburn," *Scientific American 219*, 38 (Jul 1968).

de Langre, Jacques, *The First Book of Do-In*, Happiness Press, 1607 North Sierra Bonita Avenue, Hollywood, CA 90046, 1971.

Dreisbach, Robert H., *Handbook of Poisoning*, Lange Medical Publications, Los Altos, CA, 1969.

Duff, Karl J., *Martial Arts & the Law*, Ohara Publications, Inc., Burbank, CA, 1985.

Duplaix, Nicole, "Fleas, the Lethal Leapers," *National Geographic*, Vol. 173, No. 5, May 1988, pp. 671–694.

Gleason, Gosseln, and Hodge: *Clinical Toxicology of Commercial Products,* Williams and Wilkins Co., Baltimore, MD, 1963.

Granger, Sylvia, *How to Make Your Own Moccasins*, J.B. Lippincott Company, New York, 1977.

Grant, J. C. Boileau, *Grant's Atlas of Anatomy*, The Williams & Wilkins C., Baltimore, MD, 1972.

Gray, Brian, "Dit Da Jow: Making Kung-Fu's Liquid Gold," *Inside Kung Fu,* Vol. 19, No.10, October, 1992.

Gray, Brian, "Liquid Gold or Fool's Potion?" *Inside Kung Fu*, Vol. 19, No. 7, July, 1992.

Grossman, Marc, O.D. and Cooper, Rachel, *Magic Eye:How to See 3D*, Andrews and McMeel Co., Kansas City, MO, 1995, ISBN 0-8362-0467-0.

Hatsumi, Masaaki and Chambers, Quinton, *Stick Fighting*, Kodansha International Ltd., New York, 1981, ISBN0-97011-475-1.

Hayes, Stephen K., *The Ninja and their Secret Fighting Art*, Charles E. Tuttle Company, Inc., Rutland, VT, 1981.

Hayes, Stephen K., *Warrior Ways of Enlightenment*, Ohara Publications, Inc. Santa Clara, CA, 1981.

Kreighbaum, Ellen and Barthels, Katherine M., *Biomechanics*, Macmillan Publishing Co., NY, 1990.

Lee Ying-arng, *Lee's Modified Tai Chi for Health,* Unicorn Press, P.O. Box 2448, Hong Kong, no date.

McArdle, W.D., Katch, F.I., and Katch, V. L., *Exercise Physiology*, Lea & Febiger, Philadelphia, PA, 1986.

The Merck Manual of Diagnosis and Therapy, 16th Edition, Merck Research Laboratories, Rahway, NJ, 1992.

Peppard, Harold M., M.D., *Sight Without Glasses,* Blue Ribbon Books, Inc., Garden City, NY, 1940.

Ratti, Oscar and Westbrook, Adele, *Secrets of the Samurai*, Charles E. Tuttle Company, Inc., Rutland, VT, 1973.

Rudofsky, Bernard, "The Fashionable Body," *Horizon*, Vol. XIII, No. 4, Autumn, 1971.

Stedman's Medical Dictionary, The Williams & Wilkinson Co., Baltimore, MD, 1966.

Todd, M.D., Gary Price, *Nutrition, Health, & Disease*, Whitford Press, West Chester, PA, 1985.

US Army Field Manual, Dorset Press, New York, NY, 1991.

US Government Printing Office. *Code of Federal Regulations*, Vol. 29. §1910.24, US Government Printing Office, Washington, DC, 1985.

Webster's New International Dictionary, C & C Meriam Company, 2nd Edition.

White, George M., *Craft Manual of the North American Indian Footwear*, George M. White, P.O. Box 365, Ronan, MT, 59684, 1969.

Wilhelm, Richard (translator), *The I Ching*, Princeton University Press, Princeton, NJ, 1969.

Author's Background

Robert Chuckrow holds a Ph.D. in experimental physics, which he received from New York University in 1969. He has taught physics at New York University and The Cooper Union and currently teaches physics at The Fieldston School in Riverdale, New York.

Chuckrow has been a T'ai-Chi Ch'uan practitioner since 1970 and has studied T'ai Chi under the late Cheng Man-ch'ing, William C. C. Chen, and Harvey I. Sober. He has studied I Liq Ch'uan with Sam Chin Fan-siong, Ninjutsu with Kevin Harrington, Kinetic Awareness with Elaine Summers, and Healing and Reevaluation with Alice Holtman. He has taught T'ai-Chi Ch'uan extensively and has written three other books: *The Tai Chi Book*, *Historical Tuning of Keyboard Instruments*, and *The Intelligent Dieter's Guide*. His *The Tai Chi Book* was an Independent Publisher Book Awards finalist in health/medicine in 1999.

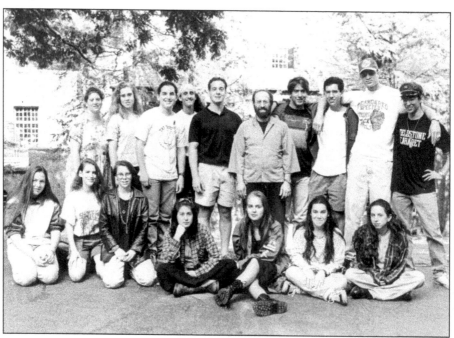

The author with some of his T'ai-Chi students at The Fieldston School in 1993.

photo by Ruth Chuckrow

Index

6 HEALING MOVEMENTS
101 REFLECTIONS ON TAI CHI CHUAN
108 INSIGHTS INTO TAI CHI CHUAN
ADVANCING IN TAE KWON DO
ANALYSIS OF SHAOLIN CHIN NA 2ND ED
ANCIENT CHINESE WEAPONS
ART OF HOJO UNDO
ARTHRITIS RELIEF, 3RD ED.
BACK PAIN RELIEF, 2ND ED.
BAGUAZHANG, 2ND ED.
CARDIO KICKBOXING ELITE
CHIN NA IN GROUND FIGHTING
CHINESE FAST WRESTLING
CHINESE FITNESS
CHINESE TUI NA MASSAGE
CHOJUN
COMPREHENSIVE APPLICATIONS OF SHAOLIN
   CHIN NA
CROCODILE AND THE CRANE: A NOVEL
CUTTING SEASON: A XENON PEARL MARTIAL
   ARTS THRILLER
DESHI: A CONNOR BURKE MARTIAL ARTS THRILLER
DIRTY GROUND
DR. WU'S HEAD MASSAGE
DUKKHA REVERB
DUKKHA, THE SUFFERING: AN EYE FOR AN EYE
DUKKHA UNLOADED
ENZAN: THE FAR MOUNTAIN, A CONNOR BURKE MARTIAL
   ARTS THRILLER
ESSENCE OF SHAOLIN WHITE CRANE
EXPLORING TAI CHI
FACING VIOLENCE
FIGHTING ARTS
FORCE DECISIONS: A CITIZENS GUIDE
FOX BORROWS THE TIGER'S AWE
INSIDE TAI CHI
KAGE: THE SHADOW, A CONNOR BURKE MARTIAL ARTS
   THRILLER
KATA AND THE TRANSMISSION OF KNOWLEDGE
KRAV MAGA: WEAPON DEFENSES
LITTLE BLACK BOOK OF VIOLENCE
LIUHEBAFA FIVE CHARACTER SECRETS
MARTIAL ARTS ATHLETE
MARTIAL ARTS INSTRUCTION
MARTIAL WAY AND ITS VIRTUES
MASK OF THE KING
MEDITATIONS ON VIOLENCE
MIND/BODY FITNESS
MUGAI RYU
NATURAL HEALING WITH QIGONG
NORTHERN SHAOLIN SWORD, 2ND ED.
OKINAWA'S COMPLETE KARATE SYSTEM: ISSHIN RYU
POWER BODY
PRINCIPLES OF TRADITIONAL CHINESE MEDICINE
QIGONG FOR HEALTH & MARTIAL ARTS 2ND ED.
QIGONG FOR LIVING
QIGONG FOR TREATING COMMON AILMENTS

QIGONG MASSAGE
QIGONG MEDITATION: EMBRYONIC BREATHING
QIGONG MEDITATION: SMALL CIRCULATION
QIGONG, THE SECRET OF YOUTH: DA MO'S CLASSICS
QUIET TEACHER: A XENON PEARL MARTIAL ARTS THRILLER
RAVEN'S WARRIOR
ROOT OF CHINESE QIGONG, 2ND ED.
SCALING FORCE
SENSEI: A CONNOR BURKE MARTIAL ARTS THRILLER
SHIHAN TE: THE BUNKAI OF KATA
SHIN GI TAI: KARATE TRAINING FOR BODY, MIND, AND
   SPIRIT
SIMPLE CHINESE MEDICINE
SIMPLE QIGONG EXERCISES FOR HEALTH, 3RD ED.
SIMPLIFIED TAI CHI CHUAN, 3RD ED.
SUDDEN DAWN: THE EPIC JOURNEY OF BODHIDHARMA
SUNRISE TAI CHI
SUNSET TAI CHI
SURVIVING ARMED ASSAULTS
TAE KWON DO: THE KOREAN MARTIAL ART
TAEKWONDO BLACK BELT POOMSAE
TAEKWONDO: A PATH TO EXCELLENCE
TAEKWONDO: ANCIENT WISDOM FOR THE MODERN
   WARRIOR
TAEKWONDO: DEFENSES AGAINST WEAPONS
TAEKWONDO: SPIRIT AND PRACTICE
TAO OF BIOENERGETICS
TAI CHI BALL QIGONG: FOR HEALTH AND MARTIAL ARTS
TAI CHI BOOK
TAI CHI CHIN NA: THE SEIZING ART OF TAI CHI CHUAN
TAI CHI CHUAN CLASSICAL YANG STYLE (REVISED
   EDITION)
TAI CHI CHUAN MARTIAL APPLICATIONS, 2ND ED.
TAI CHI CONNECTIONS
TAI CHI DYNAMICS
TAI CHI QIGONG, 3RD ED.
TAI CHI SECRETS OF THE ANCIENT MASTERS
TAI CHI SECRETS OF THE WU & LI STYLES
TAI CHI SECRETS OF THE WU STYLE
TAI CHI SECRETS OF THE YANG STYLE
TAI CHI SWORD: CLASSICAL YANG STYLE
TAI CHI THEORY & MARTIAL POWER, 2ND ED.
TAI CHI WALKING
TAIJIQUAN THEORY OF DR. YANG, JWING-MING
TENGU: THE MOUNTAIN GOBLIN, A CONNOR BURKE
   MARTIAL ARTS THRILLER
TRADITIONAL CHINESE HEALTH SECRETS
TRADITIONAL TAEKWONDO
WAY OF KATA
WAY OF KENDO AND KENJITSU
WAY OF SANCHIN KATA
WAY TO BLACK BELT
WESTERN HERBS FOR MARTIAL ARTISTS
WILD GOOSE QIGONG
WISDOM'S WAY
WOMAN'S QIGONG GUIDE
XINGYIQUAN, 2ND ED.

continued on next page . . .

DVDS FROM YMAA

more products available from . . .

YMAA Publication Center, Inc. 楊氏東方文化出版中心

1-800-669-8892 • info@ymaa.com • www.ymaa.com

Printed in the USA
CPSIA information can be obtained
at www.ICGtesting.com
JSHW060041150824
68134JS00028B/2589